Surely Goodness and Mercy
A Journey into Illness and Solidarity

By Murphy Davis

Forewords by Jürgen Moltmann and Bryan Stevenson

Peace and Justice
♡ *Murphy Davis*

Open Door Community Press
Baltimore, MD

To purchase additional copies of

Surely Goodness and Mercy
A Journey into Illness and Solidarity

phone, email, or send an order in writing to:

The Open Door Community
P.O. Box 10980
Baltimore, MD 21234-0980
404-290-2047
opendoorcomm@bellsouth.net

©2020 by Open Door Community Press
All rights reserved
Published 2020
Printed in the United States of America
ISBN: 978-0-578-66533-7

Cover: John August Swanson (1938–)
Psalm 23, 2010.
Serigraph, 22" x 30"

Author photo by Alison Reader, Framing Faces

Edited by Joyce Hollyday
Layout and design by Barbara Segal

For Ed and Hannah, who have walked with me every step of the way with love, encouragement, humor, and hope

Contents

Acknowledgments

This book was written in fits and starts over a period of 25 years. So many people have been a part of it that it is impossible for me to remember and thank everyone. Please know how grateful I am for the entire process and for everyone who lent a hand.

The members of the Open Door Community over those years included countless women, men, and children, and the community as a whole provided me a home where I could be rooted and do the work I needed to do. Most specifically, the partners and long-time members gave me time, space, and encouragement to finish the task: so thanks especially to Gladys and Dick Rustay, Nelia and Calvin Kimbrough, Heather Bargeron, and Lauren Cogswell (now Ramseur). Several folks assisted me with administrative work and did typing and editing of journal texts: noteworthy are Anne Sayre, Anne Wheeler, and Julie Martin. My dear friend Mary Eastland Sinclair was a primary cheerleader throughout. The challenging task was always, as my late cousin Mary Boney Sheats, a college teacher, always said, "to apply seat of self to seat of chair."

To say that Joyce Hollyday edited the text is a laughable understatement. An excellent editor she is – but she was so much more. One of my dearest lifelong friends, Joyce was present for much of my illness and literally midwifed the project. An experienced and noted writer, she knew how to get it done and was more than gifted as she pulled me back from countless rabbit trails to focus on the task at hand. Joyce suffered with me each time we began to gain momentum on the writing only to have it interrupted by another siege of illness. Her wry humor has been memorable and salvific. May everyone who would write a book have such a wonderful companion in the task.

Most of the work was done at the Open Door at 910 Ponce de Leon Avenue in Atlanta, in the home I now share with my partner Ed Loring in Baltimore, and in the homes Joyce has shared with her partner Bill Ramsey in the North Carolina mountains and more recently in southern Vermont. For six weeks in the summer of 2012, Marie Fortune and Anne Ganley made their little lake cabin in Robbinsville, North Carolina, available to Joyce and me for a writing retreat. It was the perfect setting: writing and re-writing through each day rewarded with a late-afternoon swim in the beautiful clear waters of Lake Santeetlah and, occasionally, a dinner of mountain trout. We are grateful and will remember.

In 2018 I was awarded a Pastoral Study Grant from the Louisville Institute. This enabled Joyce and me to travel for our work together and to pay her for long hours of labor, more than we had ever imagined at the beginning. Many thanks to Don Richter, Keri Liechty, and Edwin David Aponte for this grant, which came with generous encouragement.

Generous barely suffices to describe Steve and Christine Clemens. These dear friends have faithfully supported a multitude of wonderful efforts for justice and peace over the years. I am extremely grateful that they helped to make possible the writing of this book.

My larger family has always been in the circle, encouraging if not a bit nervous about what I might say. My sister Dot was present in hospital rooms and sick rooms through the years, and my nephew Todd has been a particular encouragement in the writing.

Since all of my medical care over the years has been in teaching institutions – where for every attending physician there are several fellows, residents, and others in training – I've had hundreds of doctors. I wish I could thank them all by name, as well as all the nurses, technicians, room cleaners, food preparers and deliverers who cared for me. Dr. Amelia (Amy) Langston, my hematologist at Winship Cancer Center at Emory University Health System, stands out. She saved my life in 2004. When other doctors had given me up for dead, Amy came in with news of a clinical trial she was directing for a drug called Pozaconozole. Other drugs had not worked, and I was slipping away. Ed quickly signed the paperwork, and the next day I started to turn back from my journey to the other side. Amy has watched over me with a hawk's eye, and I am forever grateful. Though I am now in the care of wonderful folks at Johns Hopkins Hospital, Amy continues to watch over me.

I have known for a long time that I wanted to use John August Swanson's stunningly beautiful art piece, Psalm 23, on the cover of this book. I am so deeply grateful for his gift of allowing me to do that. The serigraph incorporates images of the Peaceable Kingdom as well as the journey. Two pilgrims walk barefooted and wide-eyed through the Valley of the Shadow of Death. The night is moonless, but the pilgrims carry small lanterns, and so the night is luminous. As Mr. Swanson says, "This story connects with our own lives, as we listen to those who encourage and empower others to speak out and stand against death, violence, and hate." Thank you, John.

Barbara Segal is a great friend who is a mainstay in the Atlanta chapter of Democratic Socialists of America, where I discovered her wonderful talent for layout and design. She designed several of the Open Door Community's books that are listed in the Appendix, and I'm very grateful that she took this one on, too. In the midst of working on the journal *Emerging Infectious Diseases* for the Centers for Disease Control and Prevention during the overwhelming demands of the coronavirus pandemic, she generously kept a commitment and made time to turn my manuscript into a book. Thanks, Barbara – what a gift!

Bill Hendrix at Ironmark in Baltimore has overseen the printing of our last three books from the Open Door Press. After Ed and I moved to Baltimore, we called to tell him about this book moving toward publication, and he shared the news that he had retired. But, to our great surprise and joy, he said that he would come out of retirement to oversee the printing of *Surely Goodness and Mercy*! We are deeply grateful and so happy to be working with him again.

David Payne, who moved with us from Atlanta, serves as office manager for the Open Door Community. He has helped in ways I could hardly count, and he does it all with an amazing, willing spirit. Thanks also to Nancy L. Buc, Nibs Stroupe, Mary Sinclair, and Bill Ramsey for reading the manuscript and making helpful suggestions.

There would have been no story to tell without my Ed and our daughter, Hannah. Since the first moments of my awful diagnosis and expectations of a very short survival, they have never missed a beat. They have never taken grim medical predictions at face value, and time and again they have literally pulled me back from the thin line between life and death. If you are going to be critically ill, you must have someone to accompany you. This is not optional. Ed has literally never missed a medical appointment with me, and his accompaniment has kept me from forgetting crucial instructions and medical regimens – an ongoing risk, especially during my experiences of "chemo brain" and assaults of excruciating pain – or from losing hope.

Hannah found her vocation growing up in hospitals. She is a professor at the University of Maryland School of Nursing in Baltimore. She learned from my days at Grady Hospital in Atlanta how to advocate with doctors, nurses, and the pharmacy when I was in danger of falling between the cracks. Heaven help anybody who gets in her way when she is caring for her mama. At the most critical junctures, she has been fully present – in spite of other full-time responsibilities – and she has prevented countless disasters. To say that she has saved my life time and again is no exaggeration. And she and Ed have helped me to find something to laugh about at the worst of times.

And so it is to Ed and Hannah that I dedicate this work. The depth of my gratitude will never be known. They are my heart. As the African philosophy of Ubuntu says, "I am because we are."

Psalm 23

Adapted by Murphy Davis

Oh, my Beloved Friend,
you are my shepherd.
In your care I have everything I need.

You open the gate to green pastures.
You teach me Sabbath
and give me time to rest.
Beside the flowing stream
and the still lake
you restore me to myself in your image.

You lead and accompany me
into the path of justice and solidarity,
and I find my integrity in your way.

Even though I walk through
the valley of the shadow of death,
I am not afraid,
because you never leave me
and your love casts out fear.

With a shepherd's rod and staff,
you guide me and give me
comfort and strength.

You invite me to a bountiful table,
where enmity and divisions fall away.
"Justice is important, but supper is essential."*

You welcome me as an honored guest.
My joy overflows like a cup
poured full and always
spilling over.

Surely goodness and mercy have
run after me my whole life long.
And so I will live under the shelter of your wings
and enjoy you forever.

*Ed Loring's mantra, repeated often

Foreword

On a rainy evening in November 1983, I visited 910 Ponce de Leon Avenue in Atlanta, Georgia, and found the Open Door Community. The gathered members greeted me with civil rights songs, which Murphy Davis accompanied on the piano. I began to admire the radicality of Murphy and her life partner, Ed Loring.

In the years since, I visited the Open Door as often as I went to Atlanta – and I went rather often to give theological lectures at Emory University's Candler School of Theology. I read the community's newspaper, *Hospitality*, each month and pray for Murphy and Ed and the community every day. I appreciate and love this "other America," which turns jobless and homeless people and prisoners on death row into a Beloved Community. Are these not people of Jesus, poor, suffering, and near death, loved by God according to the Gospel?

Murphy has fought for her life against cancer – not only for her own life, but also for the collective life of those who, like her, are threatened with death. In her deathly illness, she felt close to those who are poor and sick, without shelter or in jail, and they felt close to her. They sang and prayed for her. She was not alone in her pain.

So her maladies lead, as her subtitle says, to the wonderful solidarity of the people of Jesus and Jesus himself. Solidarity is no one-way street; it is the reciprocal society of the Beloved Community. The Open Door Community in Atlanta was a foretaste, and a real beginning, of the universal vision of Dr. Martin Luther King Jr.

Facing rounds of chemotherapy five different times in her life, Murphy does not give up. I know a woman who found it so unbearable that she had resolved to die after her first chemotherapy. I myself was about to give up as a prisoner of war during the Second World War. The real misery of the jobless and the homeless and of people condemned to death is that there is always the temptation to give up. In the trust of the deeply insecure, solidarity is freedom. Solidarity gives them the will to live. And so this is a solidarity not

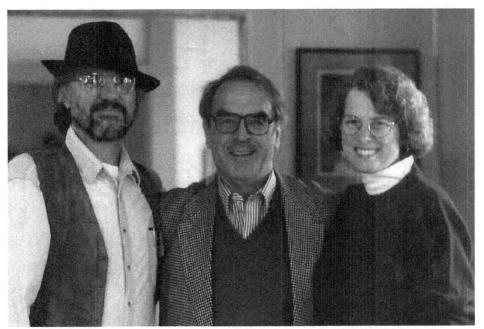

Professor Jürgen Moltmann (center) with Murphy Davis (right) and Ed Loring (left) at the Open Door Community in January 1995, just two months before Murphy's first cancer surgery. Photo by Andy Summers

only in misery, but also in the positive. The kingdom of God begins deep down in society.

The illness Murphy suffered keeps coming back, but the overcoming of illness also always comes back. Murphy is a great model for many in the struggle. "If Murphy can do it, then I can also do it," they say, and do not give up, but take hold of her courage to survive together.

Murphy has become the hope for many. She has saved many through her hard-won life. And so I close this foreword with thanks to Murphy, and thankfulness to the God of Jesus who gave us this courageous sister.

Jürgen Moltmann
Tübingen, Germany
July 2019

Foreword

My friend Murphy Davis is a free woman.

I don't mean that Murphy is outside of our destructive and predatory incarceration system; she has actually spent more time in jails and prisons than most people who have never been convicted of a crime. She is not unattached; she has been with her partner, Ed Loring, for decades and has an extraordinary daughter and wonderful family bonds. She is not unbound or unburdened; she has in fact taken on the burdens of many people in her remarkable life. She is not shielded from life's challenges and sorrows. As her beautifully written memoir gives witness, she is not immune from the devastation of catastrophic illness or suffering. And Murphy Davis is not immortal.

But she is an extremely rare free person. She lives with clarity of purpose. She has maintained an intentional ministry to the poor and condemned that can't be defined entirely by her faith and conviction, or her commitment to serve. There is something else: Murphy's soul is unchained. Her spirit fuels a keen intellect and limitless compassion to produce a kind of life force that you can sense immediately. As a powerful preacher woman, Murphy is uncharacteristically mild, sweet, and kind in demeanor – but make no mistake, she is fierce and relentless. She is "brave, brave, brave," as the civil rights folks used to say. And with this book, she has given us a remarkable new gift.

I met Murphy when I was a young lawyer in the 1980s, having just arrived in Atlanta, Georgia. The Open Door Community, of which Murphy and Ed were co-founders, was more than a homeless shelter that fed the hungry and took in those who had no place to go. It was also a place of worship, a place to congregate, and a space where we could think, talk, and strategize. I was one of the "outcast lawyers" – advocates and activists who would go there just to be present in this atypical food kitchen, shelter, church, and community in the heart of downtown Atlanta. There was something calming and comforting about the spirit of the place; I almost

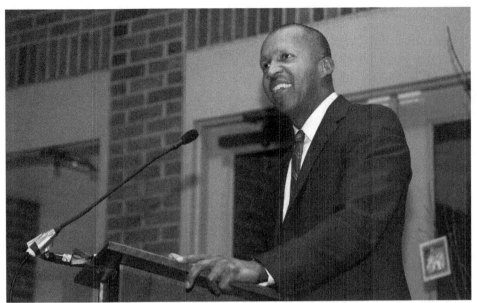

Bryan Stevenson speaking at the 30th Anniversary Celebration of the Open Door Community in January 2012. Photo by Carlton/Kari Mackey

always left encouraged. There was fellowship with the disfavored and marginalized. You'd see kindness and a commitment to the poor made real and evident in ways that made what you were doing seem connected to some larger struggle. It was very much a place striving to become the Beloved Community so many talk about but so few achieve.

Murphy has ministered to people on Georgia's death row for more than 40 years. She has been a social worker, a layperson-lawyer, an investigator, a therapist, a teacher, prayer partner, preacher, and comforter for the men and women who had been told that they were beyond hope. Something intense and unforgettable happens when you sit next to someone who has been told by their community and the established government that their life has so little value and meaning that it will be taken from them. People who are told they are beyond redemption or grace carry a unique burden that, combined with some tragic act they may have committed, can make faith and purpose seem unimaginable. Yet in this difficult space, where I first encountered Murphy Davis amidst the strain and suffering of people living under the weight of condemnation, I witnessed her unique gift for serving other people.

I saw a person with deep conviction and resolve, constantly looking for ways to bring light into dark places. She could be prophetic and reassuring, tender and uplifting. Murphy would sit with you when there was nothing to say but you just needed someone by your side. She is a stonecatcher: one who refuses to join in condemnation of the sort found in the stone-throwing crowd in the biblical story of the woman caught in adultery, but instead intervenes to catch the stones hurled by the unjust and merciless.

Murphy has power. She has the kind of spirit that could cause you to keep fighting when it was completely irrational to do anything other than submit. She made me believe things for my condemned clients, even if I'd never before seen what I was seeking. She made me believe that the prophets were right when they declared that justice must roll down like a mighty river and righteousness like an ever-flowing stream. Her conviction and her unwavering faith will be her legacy for me.

Murphy has never been afraid to ask hard questions. She has the curiosity of a theologian who does not settle for simple, incomplete answers. She has a brilliant mind that never rests on easy platitudes. She is about the truth: the powerful, life-giving, transformational truth; the kind of truth that can set you free.

We will all know illness. We will not escape suffering, pain, and some measure of anxiety and fear when our bodies start to fail, or the bodies of those we care about are in distress. We have shelves and libraries full of books with detailed descriptions about the medical challenges created by illness and injury. We can go online and find multiple sources of information to both calm and fuel our anxieties and fears. But there is precious little that honestly helps us understand how to cope, how to survive, how to endure the challenges of chronic illness. How do we have faith and keep perspective when we are in the midst of a medical crisis? It is an important question, if for no other reason than it is a question we must all face.

In my faith tradition, I have been taught that God's power is made perfect in weakness and that God's grace is sufficient. The scripture actually proclaims that when we are weak, then we are strong. It is a difficult concept to grasp, and an even harder teaching to implement. But in this remarkable book, there is something resonant about sickness transformed by grace into strength.

Murphy's book about her journey both affirms and inspires. She makes it powerfully clear that we are more than the bodies we inhabit or the challenges we must face.

I'm not really surprised that after enduring unimaginable illness, suffering, and many painful medical procedures, Murphy is still looking for ways to help other people. When I read the pages of this book and follow Murphy's path through tragic diagnoses and miraculous moments of relief and healing, I worry about my friend. I worry about her family and the rest of the large community of people who have come to love her. But I'm also grateful that she is speaking to us about what it means to survive, to live with sickness and disease, to endure suffering and still be free in the midst of extraordinary burdens to bear.

Murphy has been dancing with the angels for a long time now, but she still has the grace to think about the rest of us, to teach us some of the steps. What a rare and precious gift from a rare and precious person.

Bryan Stevenson
Montgomery, Alabama
October 2019

Introduction

Mystery and Miracle

The corridors of "Old Grady," Atlanta's aging hospital dedicated to serving the city's poorest citizens, were dark and dingy. Night and day flowed together in barely shifting tones of gray. I do not remember windows, though I'm sure there must have been some.

My 83-year old parents were there, having driven down from North Carolina to attend to their ailing daughter. My sister, Dot, waited with them. My partner, Ed, and our teenage daughter, Hannah, shifted nervously on their feet. The rustle of starched white coats moving quickly toward us in the darkened hall stays with me.

Bustled – that's the word. The two doctors bustled through the double doors and down the hall to the family conference room where we were waiting to receive the official medical report. Dr. Michelle Spector was in charge, and Dr. Marilyn Washburn moved as close behind her as she could.

Dr. Spector was my ob-gyn surgeon. She had been called into the operating room a week before in the early-morning hours of March 29, 1995, when I lay splayed open on a surgical table deep in the bowels of Grady Memorial Hospital. I've often wondered exactly where that room is located.

The first surgical team had found tumors in my upper abdomen and done what excision and repair they could. But there were more. So they called in the ob-gyn team. Dr. Spector removed the larger tumors – including presumably the primary one. A few days later, she presented my case at a pathology conference at Emory Medical School, where great minds and hearts were brought to bear. Pathologists, surgeons, hematologists, and oncologists assembled with their reports and collaborated on a diagnosis.

"Burkitt's lymphoma." Dr. Spector pronounced the strange words to us. What did we know of such language?

The grave faces of the two doctors communicated more than the words. No interpretive skill was required to know that the news was not good. As Dr. Spector spoke, her eyes filled with tears, and sorrow spilled its wet tracks down her cheeks. *What?* My heart reached toward her. Expecting a cold clinical report, we sat instead with a compassionate young woman who wept with the news she bore about this rare and lethal cancer.

That was the beginning of a mystery that has lived in and with me ever since. It is the mystery of illness and suffering shared in compassion – and then transformed from the unbearable into that which must be, and therefore *can* be, borne. From the very first moment, glimpses of that transformation were already present.

We – my family and I – sat in the sparse and dilapidated room with the news. Mom and Dad, Dot, Ed, and our 15-year old Hannah. How heavy their spirits felt. How weighty was the air. *Where could the conversation begin?*

I do not remember who spoke or what was said. I'm sure there were more tears. And – as always in this loving circle – many hugs and tender touches. What I recall most vividly as I feel my way back to that moment is that the news came to us as a family. I was never, for one moment, alone.

Ed returned later that night to our home, a large building on Atlanta's busy Ponce de Leon Avenue. Since founding the Open Door Community with friends in 1981, we had lived there, sharing life with formerly homeless men and women and advocating for prisoners on Georgia's death row. Ed shared the medical report. From there, the news fanned out – to the streets, to the cat holes of our homeless friends, to prison cells and dormitories, to homes, to churches and synagogues, to monasteries and mosques. Across the city, across the country, and across the seas.

But even before the news spread, the prayers had commenced. And the prayers have never ceased. I can hardly begin to describe what this feels like and means to us. In spite of all the crises and diagnoses and predictions of death, I am alive and well. This is simply a mystery. And a miracle.

I have no formula to share. There is no way to explain why I have lived through the impossible: a quarter century of intensive medical treatment, nine major surgeries, five regimens of chemotherapy and two of radiation, lymphoma, breast and squamous cell cancers, and a nearly fatal case of fungal pneumonia. I have often straddled the thin and precarious line between life and death.

But I am a living witness to the healing miracle of brilliant, skilled, and compassionate medical treatment combined with the daily reality of being carried through it all by prayer and hope. I have received the tender care of friends and family, nurses and technicians, doctors and hospital room cleaners, co-workers and strangers. I have been buoyed by the prayers of the faithful and the hopes of agnostics, by the persistent petitions of family and the determined conviction of poor neighbors and death-row prisoners. What an inestimable gift – to be saved by the prayers of the poor!

I want to state clearly from the beginning that I am alive not because I, and those who have helped to carry me, have more faith, or better faith, than others who have prayed and hoped for recovery. During the same years that I have survived several episodes of critical illness, many friends and family – saints all – have died, including my parents, Ed's parents, and close friends Patsy Morris, Frances Pauley, Lewis Sinclair, Mary Ruth Weir, and Mike Vosburg-Casey. Most passed on at the end of long and happy lives. Others whom I have loved, and for whom I have prayed, had their lives cut short by disease, deprivation, accidents, and exposure – and by electric chairs and lethal needles.

Why does one person live, and another facing a similar circumstance die? I do not know, and I will not presume to speculate. Some things we can know with something approaching certainty, and some things will forever remain a mystery. As the old hymn affirms, "We'll understand it better by and by."

What I have to share is not metaphysical ponderings but my story. This book is an effort to bear witness to the deep and holy solidarity that has been extended to me. I have written it with the intent to give you, the reader, a gift of accompaniment on your life path. I offer it with the hope – always – that we as a people might grow toward the solidarity that makes us each and all more human and leads us to engage actively in the justice struggle, on the path toward the Beloved Community.

Thank you for joining me on the journey.

1

How It Began

It all started in my head. December 1994 was the typical mad dash before Christmas at 910 Ponce de Leon Avenue, our two-story, 64-room home in downtown Atlanta. As holiday generosity overtook the city, donations of food and clothing poured into the Open Door Community. The large Christmas tree in our dining room, where we served lunch every day to as many as 150 people off the streets, was decorated with ornaments and angels crocheted by our friends imprisoned on Georgia's death row. At night homeless friends huddled on our porch or slept in our yard, trying to keep warm in the raw weather as we distributed blankets, warm socks and gloves. Five mornings a week, we got up in the cold predawn to cook a huge pot of grits, hard-boil 20 dozen eggs, and slice a mountain of oranges in our industrial kitchen for the breakfast we served at Butler Street C.M.E. Church.

I was frantically collecting items for the packages we would deliver to the men on death row – notebooks and pens, cookies, nuts, peppermints, and a warm hat – in hopes of infusing a bit of festive spirit into their cold, drab cellblocks. I had begun this tradition two decades before, when my work with the Southern Prison Ministry put me in regular contact with a couple dozen prisoners that I knew would not receive anything at Christmas from family or friends. It seemed like a good idea at the time. It was still a good idea. But sometime in the intervening years an assistant warden at the prison had told the men on death row that they *all* could receive a package from me. Now I was scrambling to pull together 120 of them.

Amid the flurry of activity, I felt a sinus infection coming on – an all-too-common experience for me. No time to stop, so I called a physician friend and described my symptoms. He wrote a prescription for an antibiotic.

Then came the fatigue. I had known way too much about getting overly tired. All of my adult life I had made a habit of embodying that interesting phrase "burning the candle at both ends." My general pattern was to work frenetically until I completed some task or event and then – when there was time – to crash. I could generally catch up on my sleep and be ready to go again.

But this time was different. I made it through our beautiful community candlelight service on Christmas Eve, turkey and all the trimmings served to 250 people on Christmas Day, and the usual family gatherings. Then I took a deep breath, grateful for some time to "catch up" after the holidays. But I couldn't stop sleeping. Twelve hours at a time – and then I would drag myself out of bed, still feeling heavy with exhaustion.

Wow, I thought, *I sure wore myself out this time.* Haunted by a fatigue unlike any I had ever known, I plodded heavily through January of 1995. The nurse practitioner at the Central Presbyterian Clinic prescribed another round of antibiotics. I was getting nowhere, except back around to utter exhaustion.

In February, my partner Ed Loring and I were on our annual winter visit to Warren Wilson College in the mountains of western North Carolina, teaching and reconnecting with friends cultivated over the years. I had always experienced it as a slice of joyful respite, but that year it felt a little too much like home – in the sense that it was becoming one more place where we would walk in the door and find people who wanted from us almost more than we could give. We were in back-to-back meetings and classes, and I was feeling beat up by the schedule.

But my discomfort went far deeper. I wrote in my journal during that time, "Something is badly wrong with my life, and something is going to have to happen to make me face it." Little did I know at the time how terribly true those words were.

My exhaustion continued. An X-ray revealed that there was no sinus infection. I began to question my own perceptions.

By early March, it all grew even stranger. I began to lose vision in my right eye. With each episode lasting for a minute or more, I had the sensation of a translucent veil creeping across my eye – blocking vision but not light. I was definitely in denial, and I thought of a-hundred-and-one excuses for this bizarre phenomenon.

CHAPTER 1

Sunday, March 5th, was my 47th birthday. The episodes were coming more frequently, and at last that afternoon I told Ed about them. He said that we needed to call our ophthalmologist, Dr. Jerry Hobson, right away. Our weekly Open Door evening worship service, featuring a guest preacher that Sunday, was just a few hours away, and I hated to miss it. "Maybe we could wait 'til tomorrow," I said hopefully. But Ed was clear and insistent. My denial had met its match in the concern of my loving life partner.

Jerry's response to Ed's call was immediate: "Meet me at my office in an hour." The drive from Atlanta out to Woodstock, Georgia, was almost that long. We quickly made arrangements for others in the community to take over our duties in worship leadership. The text that Sunday, the usual reading for the first Sunday of Lent, was the story of Jesus being driven into the wilderness and tested. Printed as a Call to Worship on the front of our worship bulletin, I noted before leaving, was Psalm 91, which offered comforting words in a scary and uncertain moment:

> *Whoever goes to the Holy One for safety,*
> > *whoever remains under the protection of the Almighty,*
> > *can say to God,*
> *"You are my defender and protector. You are my God; in you I trust."*
> *...And so no disaster will strike you,*
> > *no violence will come near your home.*
> *God will put angels in charge of you to protect you wherever you go.*
> *They will hold you up with their hands to keep you from hurting your*
> > *feet on the stones.*
> *You will trample down lions and snakes, fierce lions and*
> > *poisonous snakes.*
> *God says, "I will save those who love me*
> > *and will protect those who acknowledge me as their defender.*
> *When they call to me, I will answer them;*
> > *when they are in trouble, I will be with them.*
> *I will rescue them and honor them.*
> *I will reward them with long life; I will save them."*
> (Good News Version, adapted)

I tried to believe those words.

Jerry hurriedly opened up his office, accepting our gratitude and brushing aside our concern about interrupting his Sunday afternoon. I felt better in the anticipation of finding some answers about my strange symptoms. Peering into my eyes with his lights and instruments, he declared that I had "transient monocular blindness." He suspected a clogged carotid artery, a potential blockage of blood flow to my brain. "You need to have this checked by a neurologist," he said. "I think you're having a stroke warning. Perhaps a TIA" – a transient ischemic attack, or mini-stroke.

That hardly seemed possible. I had eaten lots of vegetables and very little meat over the years in order to avoid just such a reality. I remember hissing to myself, *If I have a clogged carotid artery, then why in the world did I eat all those carrots?* When we got back home to the Open Door, I celebrated my birthday with my community, defiantly downing a huge slice of German chocolate cake iced in buttery coconut-pecan frosting without a second thought.

Bright and early Monday morning, March 6th, Ed and I began our long vigil at Grady Memorial Hospital. We appeared at the Urgent Care Clinic and were immediately sent to "Investigations" for a Grady card. Grady patients must at all times carry a card that indicates their designation of expectation for payment. Options spanned the spectrum from "full pay" (designated by an "A," as I recall), to the "zero card," indicating no capacity to pay for services rendered.

Since we lived off of donations, and none of us earned a salary or carried health insurance, Open Door Community members were generally accepted as "zero card" patients. The process of getting my Grady card took three hours. "It's the price you pay," declared Ed. "Rich people pay with money; poor people pay with time."

We returned to the Urgent Care Clinic, the place you start if your needs are less critical than a heart attack or a gunshot wound. We sat there from 11 o'clock in the morning until my name was finally called to see a doctor sometime around 8 o'clock that evening. *Urgent, indeed.* I surely count as one of my best resources in this life my love of irony.

About 80 of us at any given time were stuffed into the windowless waiting room, where the air sat on all of us like the sturdy matron sat on the chair next to mine. Everybody seemed to be sneezing, coughing, hacking, wheezing, blowing, limping, and/or crying as we sat, slumped or curled on our blue plastic chairs – those of us who were lucky enough to have them. Another method of payment for Grady care is sharing the germs.

We were infants to octogenarians, and the average wait was eight hours. The room felt like a prison of sorts. We made small talk and wisecracked about the length of the wait and grumbled, while overworked staff behind a high desk refused to make eye contact when we asked them questions.

I spent most of that day with my head leaned on Ed's shoulder, sleeping like a rock. But I learned during the stretches that I was awake that other talk was going on. Many Grady patients are elderly African Americans, and they, more than any others, established the waiting-room culture. Their conversations were sprinkled generously with expressions of faith.

"Yeah, honey, I'm feelin' *real* bad, but I *know* God's gonna make a way for me somehow."

"I'm thankful that He woke me up this morning in my right mind."

"Oh, I'm *blessed*" was a frequent response to an inquiry of "How are you?"

These – the people who of all who populate our city have the hardest lives – these are the faithful ones whose mouths and hearts are filled with gratitude and hope.

And recipes. Faith and food were the two most common topics of conversation in that waiting room. "...Well, then I simmer all that in some butter with a little salt and pepper, and then that's the best eatin' you gonna find."

"Baby, don't give me none of that stuff outa' the can! I cook my black-eyed peas *fresh* with smoked turkey neck. Yeah! That's what I do. And hot sauce."

We had come to Grady and taken our seats among the poor and disabled, and we found a banquet of praise.

A couple who worked as waiters in a local restaurant spent the day "cooking" in the chairs on the other side of me from the sturdy matron. They started with Cajun food, the cuisine of the man's native Louisiana. I balked only at their imaginary production involving boudin – blood sausage. They moved from it to every possible meat, fruit, vegetable, and carbohydrate – how they dress that bird all down, put it in the oven, at what temp and with what potatoes or carrots or onions...

I could smell that food in my imagination. These new friends, companions on the waiting journey, spread a feast fit for royalty before us all to enjoy. When one course was finished, another began – before the dishes had even been cleared away. There was, in fact, no clean-up, no pots and pans to wash. The meal was free in every way. I thought of Jesus' parable of the great dinner recorded in the 14th chapter of the Gospel of Luke. Those of us huddled desperately in a crowded hospital waiting room were transformed into that great biblical throng of poor, sick, and marginalized folk streaming from all directions to feast and be filled at The Welcome Table.

Grady Memorial is a teaching hospital affiliated with the Emory University healthcare system. Years earlier, I had seen a quote from an Emory physician who referred to Grady patients in an article as "a wealth of clinical material not available elsewhere to Emory." I think that his particularly malignant attitude was unusual. But I discovered that among the many caring and committed doctors at Grady, there are indeed some who view Grady patients as their learning material – those on whom they practice before going out to perform "real" medical care, apparently defined by the exchange of money.

As I sat in that stuffy room and watched the doctors come and go, I asked myself at one point, *Why is that 12-year-old wearing a white coat?* I was in no mood that day to be some kid's opportunity for learning. I began to pray: "O God, when they call me, please let me get a grown-up." I wanted – I needed – help. But then, I reflected, didn't all of us who were sitting in that crowded room desperately need help? Wouldn't every person there have gone someplace where they would have been given more respect and faster care if they had had the money or health insurance to afford it? Grady is a last resort – a "safety net" hospital, as they say.

Finally, help arrived. A kindly, turbaned Sikh doctor asked me many questions and listened carefully and attentively. He was definitely a grown-up – and a lovely, compassionate grown-up at that! He agreed with Jerry Hobson: My vision problem might well be a stroke warning. I needed a CAT scan of my head and neck. He wrote the order for the scan, along with a referral to the Neurology Clinic. Then he wished us well and said goodnight as he moved on to the next patient. I wondered how late into the night he and his colleagues would labor before their "day's work" was done.

Ed and I proceeded to the desk to check out. The clerk took my paperwork and referrals and said, "Okay, goodnight."

Confused, I said, "But where do I go for the CAT scan?"

"Oh," she said, "in about two weeks you'll get an appointment slip in the mail, and then you'll come in about two weeks after that."

What?! Ed and I were trying very hard to take this in. My brain was foggy, but this insanity pulled it into sharp focus. "Do you mean to tell me" – I was trying not to raise my voice, but it was trembling with emotion – "that the doctor thinks I'm having a stroke warning, and you're telling me to go home and sit on my hands for a month waiting for a CAT scan?"

"This is how we do it, honey," she responded, with emphasis to equal mine.

I learned that night – and I learned it well – that excellent care is available at Grady Memorial Hospital. But there are times and circumstances in which you get to that care only if you have enough skill or education to understand what is going on and enough chutzpah to work the system. Perhaps this is true of all healthcare systems. Lesson One: You'd better learn early to be in charge of your own care.

I manipulated the system consciously and unabashedly. I took the appointment requisition into my own hands, literally and figuratively. "Where are the CAT scans done? And what time does the office open?" The clerk rolled her eyes, handed me the paperwork, and told me what I needed to know.

Information in hand, Ed and I presented ourselves at the Imaging Center on Butler Street the next morning at 8 o'clock sharp. I produced my requisition slip and listened to a gentle fuss. The receptionist muttered to herself, "What are they doing? They *know* we don't do it this way." Then looking up at us, she sighed and told us to take a seat. In an hour and a half, I was through the tube and out. The results, I was told, would be available in two days. I went home and slept the rest of that day and all day Wednesday.

Thursday morning we were back at the clinic first thing. "Why are you back here?" the receptionist wanted to know. When I told her I had come for the results, she frowned but let us wait. In a mere two hours, young Dr. Kenney was looking at me with deep concern. "We're going to admit you," he said bluntly. "I'm afraid you're having TIAs." Admitting me to the hospital, he explained, was the fastest way to get the tests I needed. Action! Not that I wanted to be in the hospital, but I was relieved to know that answers were on the way.

Within another hour, Dr. Phil Kennedy, a neurologist, was peering into my eyes and pushing on my hands and feet. I knew I was in the care of a smart and caring doctor – one of those MD/PhDs who has a heart of gold. The man was a magician.

By 11 o'clock that night, I had been through every test imaginable – all without being admitted to the hospital. The lab had drawn what felt like gallons of blood. I had an EKG. Back at the Imaging Center, I had both an MRI to examine my brain and an MRA (Magnetic Resonance Angiography) to examine my blood vessels – each an hour or so inside a noisy metal tube, which felt to me like what it would be like on the inside of a lawn mower. Then more needles and more tubes of blood.

By the end of that day, my arms looked like those of a veteran junkie after a weeklong high. A few days later, when I was making a visit at Atlanta's women's prison, I pulled up my sleeves and told the tale. Several pairs of eyes looked at me as if to say, "Yeah, girlfriend, sure!" Made me feel like part of the prison "in crowd."

When all the tests came back, the doctors were baffled. No clogged arteries. No signs of an impending stroke or even a TIA. No explanation for my symptoms. The mystery persisted.

2

"Curiouser and Curiouser"

Our friend Marty Moran, senior physician at the Sandy Springs Pediatric Clinic and doctor to all our Open Door Community children, had been calling Ed almost daily to keep up with the drama. He suggested that I see a colleague of his who had started Emory's neuro-ophthalmology program. The next day I was sitting in a chair in Dr. Robert Spector's office while he peered into my eyes. He administered lots of tests. He, too, was mystified. Concluding that perhaps I was having ocular migraines, he put me on Verapamil, a blood pressure medication that he thought would help.

A few days later it all became, to borrow a phrase from *Alice in Wonderland*, "curiouser and curiouser." My head felt stuffed with cotton and I began having trouble with my hearing. Yet another doctor told me I was suffering from allergies that were creating sinus congestion and swollen Eustachian tubes, causing 40 percent hearing loss. Then my feet and ankles swelled up, a condition I first noticed at a family party for Ed's 55th birthday. Soon the only shoes I could get around my feet were open-toed sandals.

Once again, the docs in the clinic – this time Drs. Doyle and Fackler – scratched their heads. They referred me to the Rheumatology Clinic around the corner, where I saw the attending physician, Dr. Kathy Lynn. She listened with great fascination to my list of symptoms, left the room, and returned a few minutes later with a gaggle of other physicians and medical students. She asked me to repeat the story for them. I had the feeling that I was becoming such an interesting specimen that a competition was growing among the clinics to see which would be the first to solve this strange mystery. In the meantime, I could barely walk and was doing none too well in the areas of seeing, hearing, and breathing.

I saw Dr. Spector again that week, and his brow furrowed. He felt sure that all my symptoms were connected, but he didn't know how. "I'm completely baffled," he said. Knowing how renowned his colleague is in his field, Marty Moran commented to Ed and me, "If Spector can't figure it out, you have no appeal."

On Sunday evening, March 26th, I preached at the Open Door worship service. The lectionary text that night was the story of the bent-over woman from the 13th chapter of the Gospel of Luke. Nothing if not ironic. I was feeling so bad that I skipped supper with the community and headed straight to the upstairs apartment that Ed and I shared. I ate the food he brought to me stretched out on our bed. A few minutes after I pushed away my plate, I bent over double with abdominal pain that made me want to scream. I spent a long, terrible night moving between our bed and a recliner in the next room, unable to sleep more than a few minutes at a time.

The young resident we saw the next morning at the Grady Urgent Care Clinic was convinced and confident. "Constipation," he declared. "It's the Verapamil. It's a constipating drug." His expert medical advice: "Try a stool softener." I was more than skeptical. By the next day, I could no longer stand the pain. "Ed, I'm dying," I lamented, feeling as though it were true. "And I'll be damned if I'm going to die of constipation!"

Ed called our old friend Robin Line. He had been our physician at the Central Presbyterian Clinic for several years and was by then practicing in an Emory clinic near Northside, a suburban hospital north of Atlanta. We love Robin, and there was nobody we could have trusted more. He told us to come out immediately. I already felt better. One finger on my swollen abdomen, and he was on the trail. "Acute abdomen," he said sympathetically. "That means there is air in there where it doesn't belong." An X-ray confirmed it.

Robin called the chief surgery resident in the Grady Emergency Room and Ed and I were on our way back downtown, with him doing his best to race through Atlanta's crawling "rush hour" traffic. The ER had a gurney waiting for me, and a young resident met us. After checking me over, he said that his best guess was that I must have had an ulcer. If that were the case, he told me, the surgery would be simple and take no more than an hour and a half.

CHAPTER 2

I was elated. Finally, something was going to be *done*. It had seemed like a journey with no end and, while I didn't relish being cut, I was ready for somebody to do *something*.

Ed had asked our friend Elizabeth Dede, a long-time member of the Open Door, to drive Hannah to Grady, so that she could see me before I was wheeled away for the operation. It was a happy time, especially after an IV needle began delivering Demerol to my pain-weary body. After a goodnight kiss, Hannah was off for home and bed. She had a 10th-grade mid-term exam the next morning.

Several days would pass before my mind cleared enough from the drug haze for me to understand my situation. In the meantime, I was a tangle of wires and tubes in a narcotic-induced fog. When they weren't crying, Hannah, Elizabeth, and Hannah's friend Christina Johnson were highly entertained by me, doing their best to remember all the ridiculous things I said so that they could tell me later and laugh again. Apparently the light glinting off of Christina's braces caused me to ask repeatedly, "Why do you have jewels in your mouth?" And I never grasped that spring break had begun, asking Hannah and Christina over and over why they weren't in school.

My shared room with four beds filled up with flowers and helium balloons, including a bunch tied to the end of my bed that danced around and took on bizarre and rather disconcerting human and animal shapes in the middle of the night. Hannah and my sister Dot hung the deluge of cards I received on the window blinds, creating a solid wall of color and good wishes. I heard from literally hundreds of friends – and then friends of friends – and felt buoyed by all the good cheer and prayers that were being poured out for me.

A mob of visitors showed up. Ed and Dot grew concerned. Dot finally stood over my bed and said firmly, "Now, Murph, you're going to have to choose whether you're going to host everybody in town – and a lot of people from out of town – or use your limited energy to get well." Our dear friend Mary Sinclair, who worked with the Southern Center for Human Rights and visited frequently on death row as a paralegal, took on the role of "visitor police." Stationed in the reception area, she greeted friends, kindly explained that I was resting, and invited them to write a message of encouragement in a lovely little book she had provided for that purpose.

14

At some point I became lucid enough to ask Ed what the doctors had found during the surgery. He told me gently that they had discovered cancer.

"Where were the tumors?" I wondered aloud.

"They are thinking that the primary ones were on your ovaries."

"Wow. That's pretty final, isn't it?"

I learned only later that Ed had to choke back tears to say, "Well, we don't know for sure yet."

Even my muddled brain began to grasp that I was in deep trouble. Dr. Michelle Spector made the severity of my situation very clear to my family and me in that meeting a week after the surgery, when she spilled tears. But it took me a while to comprehend the extent of the six-and-a-half-hour surgery I had undergone and the removal of my ovaries, uterus, appendix, and a large section of my ruptured small intestine – the source of the excruciating abdominal pain. As one person explained it, I had lost "all my obsolete organs."

On April 7th, Dr. Saleh, an internal medicine resident, made a visit. She came during one of the rare moments when I was alone in those first days after the surgery. She examined my lymph nodes and paced around my bed for a while. "This is one of the more difficult cancers to treat," she eventually declared. "We don't know how we'll do it." She explained that she would be consulting with other doctors. And then she added, "You understand, don't you, that there is no cure? The best we can do is buy you some time." She told me that I could reasonably expect to live another six to 18 months. Another doctor advised me to "get my affairs in order."

In the days that followed, I pondered why I wasn't tied in an anxious, frightened knot. I expect the drugs I was on had something to do with it. But it was also the case that when death stalked me, I recognized it. Death was a powerful presence I had met again and again in prisons and execution chambers, on the streets and in the cat holes of the homeless, in the deadly decisions and unctuous proclamations of the bureaucrats of state and church.

Death did not scare me because it was already familiar to me. I knew something about what it could take – and what it could not take. And even more than I knew the face of death, I knew the abundant grace of God. It was far more powerful than the awful power that wanted now to claim me.

I had a deep and abiding sense, even then, that the technical medical prognosis was only part of the truth of my situation. And I knew that I could face even the worst-case scenario. I clung to the assurance that closes the 23rd Psalm: "*Surely goodness and mercy have run after me my whole life long*" (Ps. 23:6a). I had already experienced an overabundance of goodness and mercy, and I had no doubt that they would continue to pursue me – whatever number of days I had left.

Realizing the seriousness of the illness that had taken over my body and held me hostage to a near-certain early death did, however, arouse in me a wistful longing, and a deep ache whenever I thought about the things I was unlikely to live long enough to share. My yearning was of course particularly focused on Hannah, my beautiful, loving adolescent daughter. To this day, I cannot remember that ache without welling up in tears. How I wanted to stand by her as she finished high school and moved on to college, as she chose friends and sweethearts, perhaps married and had children of her own, as she wept and laughed in the face of life's unfolding challenges and joys.

From the very beginning of her life, I had faced the possibility of losing Hannah. She was a large baby, and she was positioned in such a way that delivering her in the usual way seemed unlikely. The midwives and nurses at the birthing center prepped me for a C-section and called in the obstetrician. He reached in with forceps and, thankfully, successfully rescued Hannah. As Ed and I welcomed our daughter, I realized that in a previous era I likely would have been in labor for days and then, short of an improbable miracle, both of us – mother and baby – would have died.

In the summer of 1987, when Hannah was 7 years old, a freak accident on my brother Mac's farm in rural Tennessee forced me to face again the possibility of losing her. She was riding safely next to Mac on his tractor when a bolt on the fender gave way, causing Hannah to be thrown under the large wheel. We rushed her in the back of our station wagon to the nearest hospital, waving a white cloth all the way to alert people that this was an emergency. Thankfully, people on that winding two-lane road understood and parted to make way for us.

Hannah had a broken pelvis. But, miraculously, she suffered no paralysis or internal injuries. She spent a week in the hospital and a month in bed recovering, but she came out of it with no lingering effects. I realize that a slower reaction from Mac's foot on the brake, or a matter of an inch this way or that, and Hannah would have died or been permanently disabled. Hannah herself reflected later that her feeling at the time of the accident was, "This is what it's like to die."

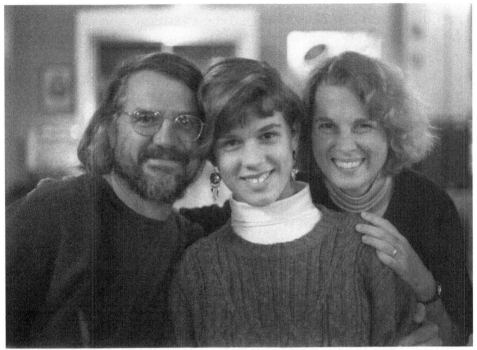

Ed, Hannah, and Murphy celebrate Hannah's 13th birthday. Photo by Calvin Kimbrough

The deep longing to be around to watch Hannah grow into adulthood was an enormous ache in my spirit. But, though it was sometimes hard to trust, I felt a clear reassurance that all would be well. The phrase that kept working its way into my heart was "There is enough."

These words had been an important affirmation for Ed and me during our years at Clifton Presbyterian Church. In 1975 Ed had taken on the position of interim pastor at the dying inner-city church. During the six years that he served there, it became revitalized around ministry with homeless persons. With another couple, Rob and Carolyn Johnson, we formed an intentional community within the congregation, and in 1979 the four of us, with several volunteers, opened the first free homeless shelter in Atlanta in the sanctuary of the church.

It was the worst possible timing. Early in that year, both Carolyn and I were pregnant. She gave birth to a daughter in May, three months early. Christina weighed two pounds at birth; I could hold her with her head in my hand and her feet at my elbow. Typical of premature babies, the under-development of her lungs was of grave concern in the following months. Hannah was born in late October. Two days later, Rob had major back surgery. Nevertheless, a week later, on November 1st, we opened the overnight shelter at Clifton. We – especially Ed – had to trust the assurance of "There is enough."

That deep trust continued as we formed the Open Door Community. We were inspired by the Catholic Worker movement, founded by Dorothy Day and Peter Maurin; by Dr. Martin Luther King Jr.'s vision of the Beloved Community; and by Koinonia Partners' long and courageous history as an interracial community in Americus, Georgia. Our witness on the streets was shaped by the Bible's prophetic tradition of justice for "the widow, the orphan, and the stranger," and our communal life drew inspiration from the picture of the early church described at the end of the second and fourth chapters of the Acts of the Apostles: "All who believed were together and had all things in common" (Acts 2:44; 4:32).

We took to heart Jesus' words recorded in Matthew 25: "I was hungry and you gave me food, I was thirsty and you gave me something to drink, I was a stranger and you welcomed me, I was naked and you gave me clothing, I was sick and you took care of me, I was in prison and you visited me" (Matt. 25:35-36). We wanted to make real in our lives his claim that whenever we did these things to the ones deemed by society "the least of these," we were in fact ministering to Jesus himself.

We wanted space to live with our homeless friends. Dr. Marilyn Washburn, a family practitioner in a Grady clinic and a Presbyterian minister with whom I had shared a couple of years at Columbia Theological Seminary outside Atlanta when we were both students, happened to know that a 64-room, former Women's Union Mission building was for sale downtown. Just right. Led by the Spirit, Ed and I sold our home, but it didn't bring enough money for the downpayment. When a couple who were good friends sold their large suburban home and bought a smaller home in the city, they generously contributed some of their equity to help us with the purchase. In July 1981 we bought 910 Ponce de Leon for $150,000. A year later, with the encouragement of Ed Grider, a friend on the urban ministry staff of the Presbytery of Greater Atlanta, the presbytery gave us

$75,000, to free us from our loan and with the thought of being mission partners and half-owners in this venture.

Not long before he left his position at Clifton Presbyterian Church for our move into the building in December 1981, Ed (Loring) preached a sermon on Jesus' feeding of the multitude with five loaves of bread and two fish. He titled it "There Is Enough." Already he had begun to preach with the cadence of a Black preacher – repeating the central phrase until the congregation picked up the chorus: "There is enough... *There is enough!*"

It became a sort of mantra for us at the Open Door Community, and many times it saw us through lean and difficult times. Usually we thought of that phrase in reference to material needs: food, clothing, shelter, money. It became the window through which we came to understand the Gospel's radical critique of capitalism, with its incessant message of individualism and scarcity: take care of yourself, save everything you can, build big houses, get lots of insurance, hoard your stuff – you might need it tomorrow.

We repeated often the words of Jesus' prayer, "Give us this day our *daily* bread." It was a petition rooted in the theology of the early Israelites, our ancestors in the faith, who relied on God to provide manna in the wilderness every day, which gave them the capacity to see "enough for this day" as a gift. God was forming them into a trusting, generous, and grateful community committed to the common good, in which all the resources were shared and no one suffered for lack of life's necessities. It was a radical notion – then as now!

Every spring at the Open Door we gathered for a Passover Seder, giving thanks for the witness of our Jewish forebears. A favorite part of that beautiful ritual of remembrance for me is the litany of proclamation, "It would have been enough for us" – in Hebrew, "*Dayenu.*" In the traditional Seder, gratitude is offered for each gift from God to the Jews: liberation from slavery, the parting of the sea, sustenance in the wilderness, Sabbath rest, the bestowal of Holy Scripture. After the naming of each, the participants proclaim, "It would have been enough for us." And yet there was – and is – still more for which to be grateful! God's gifts are abundant.

In those days after my surgery, I realized more deeply how that theology that had sustained us for so many years applied to my life. I was able to tell myself that I had experienced 47 good, full, adventurous years, rich with family, vocation, and community – a full measure of joy! There is enough.

I was not plagued with thoughts that I needed to "get somewhere I hadn't already gotten." I had been married to a wonderfully complex and creative partner for 20 years. My life, and our life together, had already been an adventure, so I was hard-pressed to complain. Our daughter, Hannah, is a delight, and I knew she would be all right without me, under the care and guidance of Ed and our community and extended family. I was not overwhelmed with worry about the future. To be spared that particular suffering was a blessing.

Still…I knew that I would fight with all that was in me to live.

3

Doing Time in the Gray Zone

As I became more conscious of my surroundings and the long road of recovery and treatment ahead of me, I was thankful for the haze of drugs that had kept me unaware for several days. My bed was in a dingy, four-bed room on 9-B, the ninth-floor surgery ward. Three televisions around me barked three different channels 24 hours a day. An NG (nasogastric) tube snaked up my nose and down my throat into my stomach, causing great discomfort. Because I needed a lot of medication, and chemotherapy affects veins, I was waiting to have a PAS (Peripherally Accessed System) port surgically implanted on the underside of my left arm for easier delivery.

My dear husband brought our Hannah to Grady Hospital for a short visit every morning before he took her to Grady High School. It was hardly convenient for them, but it was the first of many strategies and practices that Ed and Hannah undertook to keep something of a regular family schedule in the disorder of constantly changing medical regimens. At 7:40 a.m. on April 10th – five minutes before they were due to appear for their before-school visit – a transport team arrived to take me to the third floor for the PAS port surgery. I hurriedly left a note for Hannah on my bed.

Moments later, lying on a gurney in a dark room in the Interventional Radiology area, I heard a commotion in the observation room. I looked up to see Hannah and Ed grinning and waving furiously through the observation window. The medical staff let them come in for hugs and kisses, and then off to school for Hannah while I caught the next anesthetic cloud and sailed away. When I got back to my room, I found a note from my beloved daughter: "Mama, I love you so much, and hope that your arm doesn't hurt too much. Have a good day. I'll see you around 5:30,

I have algebra tutoring. Love you, Hannah." I could not have endured without such precious love.

At some point in those first days, Marilyn Washburn came by. She saw that I was in danger of falling through the cracks between the surgery, ob-gyn, and oncology services. She asked if Ed and I would like her to step into the role of primary-care physician, to help coordinate my care, and we gratefully accepted her offer.

One day a young surgery resident I'll call Dr. Chester came in and pulled out the NG tube. It was one of the greatest feelings of relief I can remember. I began to eat a little food. But before long I was launched on a frightful adventure with severe diarrhea. Lesson Two on this journey: If you're going to have major surgery and/or a serious illness – especially one that requires hospitalization – just go ahead and check your dignity at the door. Otherwise, you will involuntarily forfeit it one little chunk at a time. A *big* chunk of my dignity went down the tubes at that point.

It was bad, but it turned out to be worse for Dr. Chester. When he made his rounds one morning, I told him for the third time that I was still suffering with it. He nodded and frowned. Later that day he arrived with the full team of residents, interns, and the attending surgeon. He stood at the end of my bed and reported, as if I were not there, "The patient is eating a normal diet and tolerating it well." I raised myself up a few inches and started to protest, but they weren't looking at me or listening. I felt like a piece of "clinical material." The team turned and quickly moved on to another specimen.

When Marilyn arrived, I related the experience to her. She turned red in the face and started to fume, declaring that diarrhea in one patient could result in an outbreak in the hospital. The next afternoon I told her that I hadn't seen Dr. Chester that morning. "No," she said, handing me the letter she had written about him to the attending physician, so "hot" it nearly leapt off the page. "I think Dr. Chester might be performing surgery on the vegetables in the Grady kitchen now."

No clear sense of time existed in my world inside Grady. But after some days on the surgery ward, I was moved up a floor to 10-B: the oncology ward. Although I appreciated the improvement of having just one roommate, it was another gray zone. I had the thought when I caught my first glimpse of this new temporary stopping place that nothing had been changed from the days when this building opened its doors in the 1950s. Many a year had passed since the walls had seen fresh paint, and the long-gone painters seemed to have wielded only brushes with dull and lifeless tones. Every wall, every piece of furniture, even the air itself, was dingy. The windows were crusted with street grime.

With family and friends, I took special joy in spreading flowers and balloons around the drab ward. The altar flowers from Trinity Presbyterian Church delivered by our friend Harriet Moran decorated the nurses' station for more than a week, and a few extracted purple mums peeked over the locker of my roommate's bed. Mylar balloons perched and bobbled in the most unlikely places.

The biggest challenge on 10-B was the shared bathroom, which was down the hall. And then there was my IV pole. My arm was still attached by needles to various tubes and bags that hung from the pole, which had a bent and jammed wheel that stared defiantly at my every effort to make it budge. In that first hospitalization, I never encountered an IV pole that had a set of five functioning wheels, but this one was the worst. My mad dashes for the tiny, closet-sized community bathroom included dragging along the pole, with its broken wheel pulling resolutely against the four semi-functional ones. I tried my best to move my shrunken, post-surgical body on my spindly legs, lurching and bumping my way down the hall, praying all the way that the bathroom would be vacant. Sometimes I made it in time.

Have mercy. I had a choice to laugh or cry. Blessedly, those around me helped me to keep laughing.

The only time I had a problem with a roommate was on 10-B. She was there first, so I was the one who invaded her space. I was very weak and very sick, and though I assumed by her presence on that ward that she too had cancer, she was able to be up and around. She spent most of her time out of the bed and out of the room. Where she was I didn't know.

The main problem was her phone. In the old Grady wards, if you wanted a telephone or television, somebody had to bring it to you. I didn't want a TV, and my family didn't want a telephone there to interrupt my rest. But I had a roommate who had both in the tiny room we shared. The TV stayed on all the time and scrambled my nerves. Fortunately, I could slip over and turn down the volume when she left. But whoever called her on the phone – morning, noon, and night – had the gift of persistence. And that phone had the loudest ring I've ever heard.

Every time it rang, I jumped a few inches from the mattress. Since my roommate was usually gone, it rang and rang and rang… and rang. Once or twice, I dissolved into tears. On one of those occasions, one of the nurses came into the room. She sympathized with my jangled nerves and inability to relax.

Later in the afternoon, I was awake when my roommate came in. The tongue-lashing began before she was fully in the door. "Why are you trying to get me in trouble?" she demanded to know, claiming that she had done nothing to me. "That nurse told me off good," she continued, "like I had some kind of problem just 'cause my family wants to call me!" My heart sank. All of the chasms of race and class opened in a yawning gap between us. "I'm sorry," I stammered. "I didn't mean to make a problem for you. I'm just so tired, and the ringer on the phone is so loud."

I don't guess we resolved it very well. I am stuck with the memory of feeling like a prissy little Scarlet O'Hara whining about this and that. I hated it. I was spending my life trying to negotiate the troubled waters of racial dynamics in order to understand white privilege and move toward racial justice and the dismantling of white supremacy. But there I was, feeling stuck.

At Grady, the scriptures came alive in every moment. While I had waited for surgery, I gave way to a gunshot victim and two 11-year-old children who had been badly burned in an electrical accident. The poor and disabled, the scarred and cut, the wounded and broken – the ones whom Jesus healed – all were there. It was to such as these that Jesus proclaimed, "The Spirit of God…has anointed me to bring good news to the poor" (Lk. 4:18). It was to these that he said, "Blessed are you who are poor, for yours is the Beloved Community of God" (Luke 6:20). The people around me began to populate my prayers.

Ed named an unexpected advantage of being at Grady when he declared one day, "Well, if we had gone to Northside, we never could have gotten anybody there to come home with us." He was referring to the fact that Charles, whom we had met on ward 9-B, came to live at the Open Door when he was discharged from Grady without another home to go to for his recovery.

The seriousness of my situation caught up with me again on the oncology ward. Soon after I was moved there, I wrote in my journal:

"I have cancer and have come here for my treatment. I have come here to fight for the life that I love among the people I love. O, God, will you stay with me?"

On my first day on 10-B, Dr. Myra Rose, the attending internist from Morehouse School of Medicine, came by with her resident, Dr. Roy Jefferson. Dr. Rose had a kind and cheerful face, and Dr. Jefferson appeared with a warm smile. I liked both of them immediately and experienced those deep wells of gratitude that spring up when you know that your problems are being recognized and addressed.

The doctors came when I was alone. They closed the door and evoked the cloaked tones of confidentiality as they asked me several personal questions about my sexual history and drug use. I assured them that I had been in a monogamous marriage for 20 years and had never used intravenous drugs. The reason for the line of questioning became clear when Dr. Rose said, "Ms. Davis, we need your permission to test you for AIDS."

It all jolted into perspective, falling into place in my still-muddy brain. Burkitt's lymphoma resides in the category of non-Hodgkins lymphomas, which are becoming increasingly common in the United States. These cancers are prevalent among individuals who are HIV-positive or, more commonly, those with full-blown AIDS.

Well, I knew I couldn't have AIDS. *Could I?* I second-guessed my own confidence by wondering, *What about all the times I tended to wounds and got the blood of others on my hands before we knew about AIDS? What about our beloved dentist, who provided care for those of us at the Open Door at her own expense and was the first dentist in Atlanta to voluntarily treat patients with AIDS?* I couldn't remember ever seeing her treat anyone without gloved hands, but how good *was* my memory?

The doctors left me wondering about a lot of things, including the ever-so-slight possibility that I could find myself dealing with a devastating diagnosis of AIDS. That seemed even more difficult to bear than "just" a lethal form of cancer. I was relieved when they came back later to report a negative AIDS test. They also told me that they were going to do a bone marrow biopsy. When I looked up groggily a few minutes later, they were leaving the room. "Wait!" I called out, "Did you forget...or change your mind?"

"No," Dr. Rose chuckled. "We've done the bone marrow biopsy, and it's all over. You might be a little sore tomorrow, but you'll be fine." That was one fine dose of anesthesia.

Not long after I was moved to 10-B, I was taken by surprise one afternoon when several excited nurses appeared at my door. "What's this?" I asked.

"We're moving out," one explained. Was I condemned to a constant and unrelenting confusion? "The new ward," she continued. "The new oncology ward is ready! 10-B is closing today, and we're taking you to your brand-new room." I had become a patient at the hospital just in time to bridge the gap between "Old Grady" and the new. And the new was amazing.

The nurses rolled me out of my room – not on a gurney or in a wheelchair, but in my bed. I felt like a queen being carried down the hall, with the nurses as my court. They laughed and chattered as three of them steered my bed, one carefully guided my stuttering IV pole, another rolled the bedside table, and yet another pushed the rolling food table.

I became the first occupant of Room 1011 on ward 10-A. A single room! Everything in 10-A – *everything* – was bright and shiny and new: fresh paint, gleaming tile, sparkling new windows, and light! Light streamed in the windows; light covered the ceilings; light was in every corner. It felt like liquid cheer.

And each room had a gleaming new *private* bathroom. They were rolling us in, one at a time, and we were filling up the new rooms and halls, and our joy was infectious. The nurses had already set up the spacious and well-lit nurses' stations. Everybody – staff, patients, and visitors – *everybody* was happy.

It was a new day at Grady Memorial Hospital.

4

A Posse of Poison

A poem from my journal, for Dr. Myra Rose:

Doctor Visit, April 11, 1995

The doctor came in today
My life measured out in
*   her hands*
Days weeks and clinic visits.
Times, appointments, and occasions
*   when the poison will swarm*
*   into me*
*   to do its work*
a veritable posse
*   rounding up the bad guys*
*   and eating them up.*
Hopefully.

We make our way
*   plow our path*
Sure to know where we go
But how suddenly both
*   the path and the direction change*
How suddenly
*   life and death blur*
*   as do joy and sorrow*
*   in the tears that smear our faces*
And a poison becomes our
*   best hope.*

"Well, Ms. Davis, I have to say, you sent me to the library." Dr. Rose, the attending internist from Morehouse Medical School, was perched on a chair at the end of my bed, her head leaning lightly against the wall. "I'll have to admit, I've never dealt with a case of Burkitt's lymphoma before, so I had to hit the books and figure out a protocol. It's called ProMACE-CytaBOM, and it's going to be rigorous." I wasn't surprised. I had already been told that Burkitt's cells double in size every 30 days, making it one of the fastest-growing cancers. "I expect," continued Dr. Rose, "it's about as harsh a chemotherapy regimen as we could give you without killing you outright."

"Hmmm. Sounds inviting."

"We want to get started right away and give you the first round before we release you from the hospital."

Now her words were sounding better. *Release. Home.* Oh, how I ached to be with Hannah and Ed and our community again. Not to mention in my own bed. What a longing I had to sleep through an entire night without being waked up to have my blood drawn and temperature taken.

It was Holy Week 1995. The chemo began to drip into my veins on Maundy Thursday. That day, as with all the subsequent times I would present my arm for chemotherapy, an oncology nurse pulled a large, right-angled needle out of a sterile kit and inserted it through my skin into the PAS port. The port connected to a tube in my upper arm that was inserted into a vein that led directly to my heart, which pumped the drugs to the rest of my body. Because of the potential danger of introducing infection directly from the port into my bloodstream, only specially trained oncology staff could insert the needle and administer the procedure.

I didn't know at the time how wonderful this technology would be for me and other cancer patients. Chemotherapy typically breaks down the veins, and without such a device, finding a usable vein to administer the drugs becomes more and more difficult over time. I'm grateful to Dr. Curtis Lewis, one of the Grady physicians who helped to develop the port, who became a friend while he was head of the Department of Radiology and remained so as he became the medical director of Grady.

As I watched the different-colored drugs flow into my left arm, on their way to search out and chase away any lingering lymphoma cells in my body, I munched on crackers. One of the doctors mused,

"You might be the only patient we have who eats her way through chemotherapy."

In addition to the chemo drugs, I was on very high doses of the steroid Prednisone and Estrogen. I had awakened from surgery to discover that I had undergone a hysterectomy, among other things. Prescribing the Estrogen, one of the doctors explained, "There's no reason in the world for you to go through chemotherapy and menopause at the same time." Thank you.

As the chemo began that Maundy Thursday, I pictured my community as they gathered in front of Atlanta's City Hall that evening to remember Jesus' Last Supper with his friends, sharing the bread and the cup. Like those frightened disciples, I had to face my fear head-on. I was assured by the promise of 1 John 4:18: "Perfect love casts out fear." But what is perfect love? Was I capable of it?

I was comforted when I remembered that the Greek word *telos*, mistranslated as "perfect" in this passage, more accurately means "mature" or "full." I first learned this insight from Clarence Jordan – Baptist theologian, founder of Koinonia Partners, and author of the "cottonpatch" version of the scriptures – who has been a great inspiration for us at the Open Door. We human beings are not created to become perfect; we are taught by Jesus, the Human One, to become mature human beings. *Mature* love casts out fear. *Full* love casts out fear.

We're reminded in communion that in the bread and cup, we taste "love in all its fullness." I was struck then by the realization that "fullness" is a spatial concept. Love moves in and takes up the available space, so there is little room left for fear. As the chemo drugs flowed into me, I imagined filling up all the spaces in my body with love, crowding out the fear.

Holy Week has always been an important time at the Open Door Community. A decade earlier, we had begun keeping our annual Holy Week with the Homeless vigil, gathering each evening at 5 o'clock at a site of significance for our homeless and imprisoned friends. We held liturgies at City Hall, an overnight shelter, the city jail, and Woodruff Park in the heart of downtown Atlanta. On Good Friday we always gathered in front of the State Capitol to hear the story of the execution of Jesus the Jew, in the place where we also kept vigil every time the State of Georgia carried out a modern-day crucifixion.

CHAPTER 4

We followed the Passion of Jesus through the week, remembering his final confrontation with the powers of death, oppression, and violence; his friends' abandonment and betrayal; his arrest, trial, and execution. And we remembered – in our bodies and our hearts – the ongoing Passion of Jesus in the suffering of the homeless poor and the prisoners. Each evening after the liturgy, we commissioned a small group of people to spend the next 24 hours on the streets with our homeless friends, until the following evening's time of worship.

On the Monday of Holy Week, we always gathered on the street in front of Grady Memorial Hospital. That year, from my hospital room, Ed and I had followed the liturgy, conscious of our friends on the street 10 stories below us, as they were of us. It felt more than strange to know that this familiar vigil was taking place without us – so near and yet so far. But both we and our community carried on with the distinct work that was set before us, and the liturgy enfolded my journey straddling life and death, with the deepest hope for a glimpse of resurrection.

On Good Friday, after being kept for a day of observation after my first chemo treatment, I was released and returned home to the Open Door. "Welcome Home" signs, balloons, and flowers greeted me, and never did decorations look more beautiful to my appreciative eyes. That moment was the first of many times that I experienced the sweetness of returning to my own space, my own bed, my own clothes. I'll never forget the delights of that first night: a dark room, uninterrupted sleep with my husband, and quiet (well, as quiet as it gets on bustling Ponce de Leon Avenue). I felt gratitude at a deeper level than I ever had before for the simplest things of life, and for the gift of sharing them in the context of a loving family and community.

Soon after I arrived home, several friends quietly offered the same invitation, saying essentially, "If you need to be in a quieter, more private, more comfortable space than the Open Door to recuperate, I'm sure we can arrange something." As much as I genuinely appreciated their concern, their offers seemed preposterous to me. I had never even thought of being anywhere else.

Ed and I had a wonderful apartment at the Open Door, with everything we could possibly need. We had the built-in supports of life in community: people beyond our immediate family to help prepare food, clean, and provide physical care. And the crucial presence of others beyond the community was available to call on when the emergencies would – and did – come. But most of all, what had seemed clear from the start was that healing is a contextual discipline and gift. The large and diverse Open Door family that surrounded our smaller family had been my life's work and context. If I was going to recover, it would surely be the context of my healing as well.

In our experience, 910 Ponce de Leon had been the geography of ongoing miracles. After years of being pounded on the streets or in prison, haunted by poverty or mental illness, broken souls walked in our door and literally "came alive" again in community. Sleeping in a warm bed, eating regular meals, and being called by name brought about amazing transformations.

Barbara Schenk came to us suffering from schizophrenia, her behavior wild and erratic, her desperate moans echoing through the house sometimes all night long. When she felt comfortable and safe enough to sit down at our piano, often playing for an entire afternoon, her spirit calmed. Robert Tolbert also found respite from his mental illness at our piano and shared his beautiful gift of music with the community. When Carl Barker experienced welcome within our walls, he rediscovered his talent and began to draw stunning political cartoons for those walls and for our Open Door newspaper, *Hospitality*. We learned that in his life before homelessness, he had been a regular cartoonist for the *Chicago Daily Defender*.

Alcoholics held on to sobriety for years among us, people with mental illnesses found stability, battered souls discovered safety and peace. All of that, of course, came in the midst of daily failures and constant loss to the demons of alcohol, drugs, mental illness, and other terrors. But the failures were mitigated by these occasional but stunning miracles.

I could fill a book with the resurrection stories we witnessed. What sense would it have made for me to go away to seek healing in more comfortable physical surroundings but in isolation from this rich life that is a daily context for healing miracles? I did not know whether I would get cured of the cancer – that would unfold over time – but I did know from the beginning that I was experiencing healing.

It came in one unexpected way. The doctors had to open me all the way up for the life-saving surgery and staple me back together. A 23-inch scar running the length of my torso bears witness to the extent of their work. Because the tumor growth had caused my small intestine to burst, the prospects for infection were high. A few days after the surgery, I spiked a fever. The doctors removed the staples and reopened the wound to expose it to healing air and frequent dousings with a saline solution.

Since chemo drugs attack the immune system, and the immune system is what helps us to heal, the doctors told me that it likely would remain unhealed for the duration of my chemotherapy. For several months I would have an open wound like a trench in the center of my body. It had to be carefully tended – cleaned, examined, and re-dressed – twice each day. It was tedious, gory, and unnerving work.

Hannah stepped up to the task. It seemed a bit much to me for a 15-year-old to take on, but she was stubbornly clear about being the one to do it. She was well served by growing up in a community close to the nitty-gritty of life on the streets. At the Open Door we dealt daily with the downside of human biology and the myriad of its not-so-pretty bodily by-products. We served a constant stream of people with untreated illnesses and wounds: feet ravaged by relentless movement and ill-fitting shoes, by frostbite and gangrene; folks who had bled or vomited or soiled themselves for lack of the simple necessities of a bathroom and toilet paper, who carried layers of street grime and odor for lack of running water and clean clothes.

After many a gag reflex and more than a few tears, one either flees or has to embrace the absurdity of life and develop a rather earthy humor to deal with it all. Laughter often saved us, keeping us from being overwhelmed and paralyzed by sorrow. Our experience paid off as we faced this new predicament. Confronting and surviving a serious illness requires not taking oneself too seriously, and it helps a great deal to surround yourself with people who can help you laugh, especially at yourself.

Every morning before school and every evening before bed, Hannah washed and disinfected her hands, carefully removed my bandages, cleaned the wound, inspected it thoroughly, and re-dressed it. She was the first to spot a small infection. The doctors affirmed her diagnosis and quickly treated it with antibiotics.

This arduous task was an important part of Hannah's coping with the seriousness of my illness. It was a concrete, hands-on way to love me and help move me, day by day, toward healing. After a while she gave herself permission to spend an occasional night with friends, or let me tend my own wound on busy mornings, but she honored the commitment with all her considerable determination. Thanks to her careful attentiveness, the wound eventually did heal. And with the healing of my wound came some healing for the bruised spirit of my child.

Two days after I came home from the hospital, at the end of Holy Week, we had our usual Easter Sunday service at the Open Door. I was too weak to join the crowd of homeless friends and volunteers gathered in our front yard. But with assistance, I was able to make it out to our second-floor balcony, where I offered the benediction over the throng in my bathrobe. The pope in his ornate robe, delivering his Easter address to tens of thousands from the balcony of St. Peter's Basilica in Rome, couldn't have felt more important or appreciated.

In that season of resurrection, my faith continued to carry me. I wrote in my journal on April 20th, a week after my return home:

My faith is simple – childlike, I suppose. When I went to college, I sort of waited for doubt to set in – listened with interest and attention to accounts of angst-driven struggles and searches among peers. It never came. I wondered about myself. Was I missing something essential? Could I grow to maturity without the Ordeal of Doubt?

God is with us. A simple fact, like bedrock in my life. We live, move, and have our being in the cradle of God's Everlasting Arms.

Though I have often wondered why God was being so quiet, or when the fiery Spirit was going to show up to set things right, it was not a matter of wondering whether or not God's presence was true. It was a matter of wonder at the Truth of it. Reverence for Life itself that flows into the conviction that "Everybody's got a right to the Tree of Life."

I understood first the God of Creation. God in the ancient live oak trees of City Park in New Orleans – with the long limbs that reached down to a small child, sheltered her in their arms, and taught her to love trees. God in the creeks of the North Carolina mountains who spoke to me in gurgles, babbles, and joyful cascades. God of the majestic peaks of the Appalachians who stood in my heart's eye as strength and beauty, steady and unmoving.

It was later that I came to have some understanding of God on the jagged edge of history – the God who acts for good and for justice. The God who promises a foretaste of the New Creation in the present.

CHAPTER 4

In these days the simplicity seems to serve me well. God is my loving, attentive Creator. Life is a gift; and through the troubled waters, I am carried by God's good Spirit. I will not drown. The power of death and hell must stand back in the presence of the Everlasting Arms. The power of Resurrection Life is on my side and shows its daily presence in the loving faces of family and friends who do literally carry me through these days.

Thanks
Life
Love
Friendship
Family
The hunger and thirst for wholeness

What more?

5

The Gift of Solidarity

My first memory of Albertine Yorke is the quick, clicking sound her high heels made on the worn, polished, granite hallway floor of the Grady Hematology Clinic. The old clinic on the 12th floor of the hospital had no waiting room. We patients checked in at a window just inside the double doors, and then we sat in plastic or metal chairs scattered up and down the hallway, where we waited to be seen by the doctors.

So there we were – Ed and I – sitting in the hall. Still only a few weeks past major surgery and my first chemo treatment, I was feeling none too spiffy and surely had not arrived at the place of thinking straight. But these high heels clicking rapidly across the floor got my attention.

"Ms. Davis?" The voice lilted with a British Caribbean cadence. "Are you Ms. Davis?"

"Yes, I am. Hello."

"My name is Albertine Yorke. I am your social worker."

The words might as well have been spelled out with those little, wooden alphabet blocks with which children play. They hung there in the air as I tried to wrap my foggy brain around them. Perhaps the blocks were to be rearranged. These were strange words indeed.

"I am your social worker."

"I am *your* social worker?"

"I am your *social worker*?"

Wait a minute. Somebody got something wrong here. My brain struggled mightily to protest. I needed to think of how to explain my way out of this.

Maybe we should start over: "Hello. *My* name is Murphy Davis. I am a Presbyterian minister, and I am a pastor among people who are homeless and imprisoned. I visit frequently at Grady Hospital. I come here to accompany and advocate for the poor who are sick or injured. I often work with Grady social workers. They are colleagues. Co-workers. Peers. Is there something I could do to help *you*?"

No, that wouldn't work. But still – surely there was some mistake. Did I stammer "Yes, ma'am"?

Ms. Yorke couldn't see my internal struggle, and she hurried on to explain. "We want to explore whether we might apply for you to be qualified for Disability. I need your permission to speak to Dr. Newcom about this."

What did I say? Did Ed handle it? I have no idea. But having one way or another received my consent, Albertine Yorke hastily turned and disappeared into an examining room in search of Dr. Samuel Newcom, chief attending physician of the Emory-Grady Hematology Clinic. I was left in the hall in a state of bewilderment.

"I have a *social worker*."

"*I* have a social worker."

It all happened really rather quickly, and I was left to ponder the fact that Ms. Yorke did not find our exchange at all strange. Nor did she recognize my awkwardness and discomfort in her role with me. Over time, she became a good friend, but that day I was just another Grady patient she was determined to help.

My care had already cost thousands of dollars for clinic visits, surgery, and a long hospital stay for recovery. And I was in the midst of a very expensive chemotherapy regimen. Part of the job description of the Grady social worker is to explore any possible avenues for reimbursement to the hospital from county, state, or federal government programs for its services to uninsured patients.

I was a Grady patient: a bona fide charity case. After 25 years of coming in and out of this hospital – always in the role of…well, I hate to use the word…in the role of a *professional* – here I was. Pale and skinny and weak, I sat in that hall with the sick and the dying. And I could no more pay for my care than any of the rest of the uninsured.

Funny. I have always claimed to believe that God answers prayer. And it is true that Ed and I had been praying for at least 20 years – praying persistently and with focus – to find the path of solidarity with the poor. We had asked God to give us the *gift* of solidarity. Now I was feeling a bit unsure about whether I wanted this gift. Nope, I didn't anticipate it feeling like *this*.

In the months around our move to the Open Door in December 1981, Ed, Rob, Carolyn, and I had, one by one, given up our salaried work in order to devote ourselves more intentionally to ministering to prisoners and creating community with people from the streets. My salary was the last to go. I had formed the Southern Prison Ministry and administered the funding. From 1977 until the spring of 1982, I had compensated myself $620 per month – an annual salary of $7,440. I had hit, and then forsaken, the highest salary I would ever see. We went on from that time living off of donations from our Open Door supporters.

Until that spring of 1982, we and our children had very fine health insurance policies – Rob and Carolyn with the United Methodist Church and Ed and me with the Presbyterians. But we began to ask ourselves, *How can we strive for solidarity with and among the homeless poor while we hold onto the privileges of salary, health insurance, personal savings, and other such "perks"?*

We began to understand that if we continued our lives inside the vestiges of power, privilege, and access to the system's benefits, we would always be set apart from the sisters and brothers with whom we wanted to build community. Solidarity would have little meaning if we lived together with drastically different resources available to us. So the four of us ditched the personal financial benefits of being middle class for a new way of life. We decided that all of us at the Open Door would depend upon the care of volunteer physicians, the "charity clinics" with a sliding scale, and – for any extraordinary needs – Grady Memorial Hospital.

Grady, the only option for residents without health insurance, is the fifth-largest public hospital in the country and has one of its busiest Level 1 trauma centers. It opened in 1892 with 14 patient rooms – for whites only. The current building, opened in 1945, is in the shape of an H. It was constructed with a very long hallway between two wings facing the city for white patients and two in the back for Black ones. It's about as inefficient a medical floor plan as you can imagine, but segregation trumped good design. The hospital is still referred to sometimes as "The Gradys," particularly among older African-Americans.

Though those of us at the Open Door all took our turns going to Grady clinics for routine health matters, our commitment had remained largely an abstraction. Up until then, it had never been a life-and-death matter. But there I was, a real live Grady hospital patient, flat on my back and in dire need. Grady is the "charity" hospital – the poor peoples' hospital – *my* hospital. I didn't realize until much later how many of my middle- and upper-class friends and associates were horrified that I had gone to Grady for my surgery and treatment of such a serious illness.

But the die had been cast in 1982 with our community's decision to forego health insurance. We had restructured our lives for solidarity. We had offered fervent prayers for solidarity in the years since. And now I was practically gagging on the fruit. This was *it!* Solidarity was realized in my life, and I was not at all sure how to be comfortable with it.

To be in solidarity with the poor is to experience poverty, and one of the basic realities of poverty is powerlessness. Not having money is one thing; powerlessness is quite another. Lying in a hospital bed at Grady, or sitting on a folding chair in the hall of a Grady clinic, I had realized that my life was – no less than the lives of my poor sisters and brothers of the streets – out of my control. Though it was far more difficult than I had ever imagined, I knew instinctively that this reality would be "good for me." I did not know how or why, but on some mysterious – perhaps mystical – level I was quite clear that my life, and perhaps my death, would be richer and deeper because of this experience of powerlessness. I was getting my first glimpses of an enhanced capacity for solidarity.

For years I had preached and written about the threat of death as the common experience of the poor, whether on death row or the streets. By judicial decree, by neglect or deprivation, what we do to the poor is threaten their lives and well-being. I have been on "death watch" with death-row prisoners in the hours before their executions scores of times, and I have come to see that to be poor in this country is to be perpetually on death watch.

Gustavo Gutierrez and other liberation theologians remind us that to be poor is to be dying – living every day, every moment, in the presence of death – and in the presence of the threat of death. Before physical death comes, the poor experience the death of health and well-being, the death of power and choices, the death of human dignity, and for many the death of hope itself.

Before the development of modern industrial culture, human beings lived much closer to the daily reality of death – and most people in the world still do. But those of us in North American mainline culture live lives of segregation: the old over there in a nursing home, the mentally ill in institutions and the condemned in cells, the homeless under bridges – out of sight and out of mind. We of the upper classes intentionally shield ourselves from those whose suffering might be unpleasant to us. We do not want to watch the death of the poor.

To live in solidarity with the poor is to share proximity to death. My years on death row and with homeless sisters and brothers had taught me more about death than I ever knew to look for. The prospect of my own death joined the concerns that had become part of my life, my work, my prayer.

No one was about to kill me. No one wished me dead (well, maybe a prosecutor or two). The politics of the death I faced were different, but it was no less death. I had been told to expect death from this aggressive cancer – if not soon, then before long.

"You've been with us all these years. Now you really know what we're going through," a friend on death row wrote to me. "You are one of us," wrote another, "you have a death sentence, too." One friend expressed his hope that I would "get a stay." The cards and letters poured in quickly and often from death row, bearing expressions of sorrow, fear, love, solidarity. Many prayers were promised and offered.

Chaplain Jordan, the Muslim chaplain at Metro State Women's Prison, came to visit me at Grady. "The women made me promise," she said, "that I would come up here myself and let you know that all of us are praying our hearts out for you every day. We never gather for worship that one of the women doesn't stand to weep and pray for your restoration to health."

The good fruit of accompaniment was flowing around me in showers of blessing, as those I had been with in prison now joined me on my own perilous journey. I felt a deep communion with my friends on death row – the many who had died by execution, suicide, or medical neglect – and those on the streets who had died from exposure or malnutrition. The life-changing experience of solidarity with the poor had begun prior to my life-threatening illness, and it was a bedrock resource in a crisis.

What I felt as I faced my own death was a simple recognition that I had undeniably taken a step farther on this journey. I was grateful that I had already been well equipped to walk into this theretofore unknown – and certainly mysterious and grace-filled – territory. A new dimension forced its way into my existence, and it led me to gratitude for every day of life.

Health care, in our system of consumer capitalism, is a commercial enterprise. If then one receives it – as I have – and cannot pay for it – as I cannot – one is supposed to feel deeply embarrassed, ashamed, humiliated. Over the years Ed has often said of our life at the Open Door, "We are sophisticated mendicants." Well, now we could forget about the "sophisticated" part. We are beggars: dependents, some of the many "undeserving poor," a "drain on the taxpayers." I had to my name not one shred more dignity than that accorded to those individuals the police and businesspeople of downtown Atlanta have publicly labeled "aggressive panhandlers."

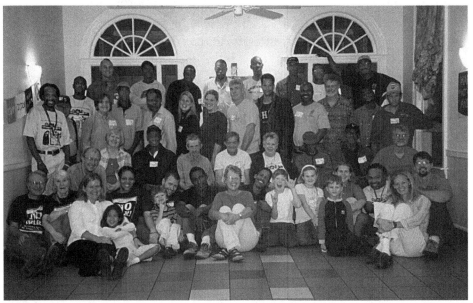

The Open Door Community and friends, Labor Day Sunday 2005, one of the annual photographs included every year in Christmas cards sent to death row and other prisoners. Photo by Murphy Davis

During that first stay at Grady, I cultivated an appreciation for, and identification with, the story of Jesus and the paralyzed man recorded in the second chapter of the Gospel of Mark. The man's friends were so determined to get him healed that they circumvented the gathered crowd, tore open the roof, and lowered him on his mat in front of Jesus. Jesus was so moved by their faith that he healed the man, who picked up his mat and left dancing and glorifying God.

I felt like that man. I had a multitude of dear family and friends symbolically tearing off roofs and carrying me to Jesus' feet for healing. In my utterly powerless state, I could do nothing but surrender to their loving, extravagant care and tireless determination.

I had learned by then that Burkitt's lymphoma – named for an Irish gastroenterologist in the British army named Denis Burkitt, who had identified it among Ugandans in 1958 – is most common in boys and young men in the low-lying areas of tropical East Africa. The tumors generally occur in the neck and jaw. There seemed to be no adequate explanation for how this middle-aged North American white woman could come up with Burkitt's tumors in her abdomen.

Allen King, a former college literature professor of Ed's and longtime friend, responded to the diagnosis, "My Gawd! The lengths to which some people will go to be *different!*" Marshall Handon, a friend and colleague through Atlanta's Concerned Black Clergy – of which Ed and I had been founding members – exclaimed at a meeting when he learned of my strange "statement of racial solidarity": "Lord, she even got a Black *disease!*" I think they waived my annual membership dues. I know that the prayers of the brothers and sisters were fervent and steady when the invitation went out to keep Ed and me "wrapped in prayer." And I was grateful for several members' visits.

I sat there in that stuffy hall on the 12th floor of the hospital as it slowly began to filter into my mind and heart: My prayer was being answered. I was – really and truly – a Grady patient, and I could not move ahead with the expectation of any special treatment or consideration. I had met my social worker.

She was not gone long. "No," chirped Albertine Yorke. "Dr. Newcom said you will *not* qualify for Disability, because your cancer is curable."

Curable danced off Ms. Yorke's lilting tongue and hung in the air. What about what the other doctors had said? What about the grim faces that had speculated a prognosis of six to 18 months? What about the somber admonition to "get your affairs in order"?

Perhaps Ms. Yorke had heard it wrong. Perhaps Dr. Newcom was confusing me with another patient. To trust these words, we would have to hear them from the good doctor himself, looking at me with the correct medical chart in hand. Curable? Indeed.

He said it. On that very day. *Curable*. "Burkitt's lymphoma is a very lethal cancer," Dr. Newcom conceded. "But if it doesn't kill you at first, it's one of the forms of cancer that is most responsive to chemotherapy. Of course it nearly killed you. But since it did not, I am expecting a complete remission of the cancer."

Sam Newcom was an attending physician with Emory University School of Medicine and a highly respected research hematologist. Ed and I sensed immediately that this was a physician to trust and appreciate. Not one for "warm and fuzzy," on that day and in days to come he always gave it to us straight, and we had full confidence in him.

He explained that the rupture of my ileum, the lower part of my small intestine, saved my life. While the surgeons were repairing it, they found and removed the cancerous tumors. The success of my case, I learned over time, was an occasion to reconsider the prevailing protocol – from using chemotherapy as the first medical response in all cases to considering surgery followed by chemotherapy as the best course of treatment.

Because of the surgery, I had begun chemo with no detectable tumors. Since no cancer cells were found in my blood, my bone marrow, or anywhere else in my body, the Hematology Clinic doctors – Dr. Newcom, Dr. Neil Marrano, and Dr. Sid Stein – expected to see me fully recovered. But they never held out any false promises. Recurrence of a non-Hodgkins lymphoma is always a possibility, if not a likelihood.

But as for the here and now, you, Murphy Davis, uninsured Grady patient – you are *curable*. You might be a charity case. You might have a social worker. You might be experiencing the hundreds of little indignities that come with a serious illness – and especially the many that come if you're dependent on charity care – but…you are curable! Though I wasn't able to leap and dance at that point like the paralyzed man healed by Jesus, my heart surely felt like it.

A serious issue was emerging in my life: Where to put all this joy? How to contain it? How to express the overwhelming, overflowing gratitude I was feeling *for every day of life*, for every person in my path, for every hint of good news, for the wellspring of hope that was there even before hearing any good news?

What shelf did I have in myself strong enough to hold this gift?

6

Letting Go

Eventually I would learn to pronounce all the strange substances entering my body that were killing the cancer and saving my life: Cyclophosphamide, Doxorubicin, and Etoposide, followed a week later by Cytarabine, Bleomycin, Vincristine, and Methotrexate, combined with high doses of the steroid Prednisone. Most entered my bloodstream through the PAS port, one by intrathecal injection through a long needle inserted between two vertebrae at the base of my spine. Each chemo cycle lasted three weeks – one week each on the two different drug regimens, followed by a week off.

The Chemo Room at Grady was around the back corner from the Hematology Clinic. We patients sat in five chairs close together. Nancy Feldman, who was in charge, brought quiet and friendly competence to a job so large that no one should have been handling it alone.

The chemo drug Methotrexate, if left in my body unstopped, would have caused damage to my heart, kidneys, and/or other organs. So after each infusion of the drug, I had to begin exactly 24 hours later to take nine tiny pills of the rescue drug Leucovorin, at 6-hour intervals for the next 24 hours. This meant setting the alarm clock to keep the schedule throughout the night and day, and it took both Ed and me to keep it straight – especially since the drugs often muddied my mental clarity. Those of us who have experienced "chemo brain" know it as a true phenomenon, and recently the medical establishment has officially affirmed our experience and verified its existence.

On one occasion we were leaving the clinic after chemotherapy, and we were almost to the door when Ed said, "Wait a minute! Weren't we supposed to get some medicine to take home?" We had nearly left without the Leucovorin. Another time we got the drug from the pharmacy and read the instructions on the label: "Take as needed." Dr. Newcom hit the roof when I showed him that prescription label.

Throughout the chemotherapy, I had many medications to take in varying quantities at different times of the day and night. Ed and I have three master's degrees and a Ph.D.-and-a-half between us, and we could barely keep it all straight. I ached for the many Grady patients who surely fell between the cracks of such complicated regimens.

One day that summer I was kicked back in the reclining chair waiting for my chemo infusion. My notebook was open to the page where I had listed the drugs for Week 2, Round 3. Nancy was busy with other patients, and another nurse who had come to help her attended to me. When she laid out the drugs on the table beside my chair, I double-checked the list. They were the wrong drugs: the same ones I had received the week before. A second dose would likely have been a lethal overdose. This episode of a near-fatal mistake repeated itself a few weeks later.

That summer of 1995, the story of the death of *Boston Globe* health columnist Betsy Lehman at the Dana-Farber Cancer Institute made the national news. She died of an overdose of Cyclophosphamide, a chemotherapy drug that was also part of my regimen. I was excruciatingly aware of how easily it could have – and almost did – happen to me. If it could happen in one of the leading cancer institutes in the world, it could surely happen at Grady.

Ed and I would come to learn through my years of cancer treatment that every step of the way brought new protocols, new technologies, and new drug therapies. It has been awe-inspiring to realize the fruits of ongoing research and testing that have benefitted me and so many others. The very first drug I was given when I started chemotherapy (and I still have a bottle in my medicine box today) was Zofran. This powerful anti-nausea drug was approved for use at Grady *the very week* I started chemo. Though I experienced some nausea, it was not the relentless living hell that others before me had to suffer through. If I had started chemo a week earlier, I would have faced a very different reality.

I had never thought to give thanks for the thousands of men and women the world over who spend their lives in laboratories searching for The Cure and all the intermediate strategies. As our perceptions broadened, so did our gratitude – and our sense that we needed to ask for forgiveness for not noticing before.

For the first three months, as I was making my way through six three-week chemotherapy cycles, I felt extremely weak and faint at points. I passed out cold once at the Imaging Clinic, hitting my head on the granite floor. None of the doctors could explain why these fainting spells were recurring. One of the good things about sharing close quarters in the chemo room is that we patients got to know one another's stories and readily shared medical information, which turned out to be a godsend.

"It's the steroids, girl," explained Laura Chastain, one of the other chemo patients. "They don't tell you you've gotta come off 'em gradually." Once I learned to wean myself in stages from the megadoses of Prednisone I was on, the fainting stopped. I tried to explain this carefully to my doctors, hoping they would value the wisdom of our experience and change the protocol for future patients.

The list of potential side effects for all these drugs could fill an encyclopedia: myelosuppression (lessened bone marrow activity), hyperuricemia (gout), stomatitis (oral inflammation), nausea and vomiting, neurotoxicity, vesicant (blisters), cardiotoxicity, gastric irritation, hemorrhagic cystitis (urinary tract inflammation), renal and hepatic dysfunction (kidney and liver failure), alopecia (hair loss), insomnia, areflexia (lack of reflex), motor neuropathy (weakening muscles), constipation, pulmonary toxicity, hyperglycemia (high blood sugar), and hypotension (low blood pressure). As if these weren't enough to worry about, I was particularly surprised to see "abnormal buttoning or writing" on the list of potential neurotoxicity symptoms. I was pretty sure I had buttoning mastered, but I had been accused more than once of writing reflections out of my experiences on death row and the streets that were considered far from "normal," and I didn't think I needed a push in that direction.

About a month after my first chemo treatment, I was sitting in our kitchen when I experienced a distinct tingling. It crept up the back of my neck and spread over the whole of my scalp. I knew right away what had happened. "Wow," I said to Ed, "my hair just let go."

"What?"

"I just felt a tingle all over my scalp. The roots of my hair just let go."

Sure enough, the next morning I woke up to find my pillow covered with small clumps of my hair. Every day more appeared – on my clothes, in my hairbrush, caught in the drain of the shower. That chemotherapy causes hair loss is fairly universal knowledge, and I was getting very heavy doses, so it was no surprise and I did not experience it as a trauma. And, as it turned out, it was the least of my problems that summer.

When Ed and I went out for dinner on May 25th to celebrate our 20th wedding anniversary, I ate a hearty seafood supper and then doubled over with abdominal pain. We drove on home, and I endured a night of nearly unbearable pain. It persisted into the next day without relief. Ed strongly encouraged me to go to the Emergency Room. None too anxious to be back in the clutches of the hospital, I waited and hoped that the pain would go away.

Finally, I relented. Our dear friend Joyce Hollyday from North Carolina had come to visit, and she and Ed drove me to Grady, where we took up the vigil in the ER. After I was finally seen by a doctor, I spent that night being wheeled on a gurney from one place to another for diagnostic tests and examinations.

Finding an available wheelchair at Grady's ER is virtually impossible, so I had arrived in ours from the Open Door. While I was having all the tests, Joyce had the role of guardian of the precious chair. As we journeyed through that long night, she was turned away from several evaluation rooms by "family only" regulations. We still laugh at the rather comical image of Joyce alone outside those rooms scattered throughout the hospital, standing guard over an empty wheelchair and then pushing it on to the next stop, all night long.

Lying on some sort of Styrofoam-like block with my head and legs draped over the edges, I had an abdominal X-ray and thought I was going to die from the pain. When the doctors determined that I had an intestinal blockage, one of them inserted the dreaded nasogastric tube. Just over a month after I had been released, I was readmitted to Grady. As I was being wheeled back on to ward 10-A in the direction of a double room, one of the nurses ran up and protested, "No, no! Room *1011* is Ms. Davis's room." Wow. Somebody had marked that room for me, and I was taken down to my old familiar digs near the end of the hall.

In the morning our faithful friends Nan and Erskine Clarke came to sit with me and help as they could. Their visit enabled Joyce and Ed, who had spent most of the night standing by my gurney in the ER, to slip home to grab a bit of sleep. Later that day my parents arrived for an already scheduled visit. I felt the presence of my Mom and Dad, of Erskine and Nan. I "saw" them, but it was as if they were in a distant land and I…well, I was out at sea. I was tethered to my spot by the IV lines and the detestable but salvific NG tube.

I spent what felt like an eternity in the bed in "my room" on 10-A. Those were days of unrelenting torment. The bellyache from hell kept pounding me with a vengeance, compounded by the hideous discomfort and splitting headache caused by the NG tube. Never again, I learned during that visit, would I let a doctor force an NG tube that was larger than a "14 French" down my throat.

I slept in small snatches and wished for the oblivion of sleep when I was awake. I remember thinking of Flannery O'Connor, the Georgia writer who has long been one of my favorites. During her years of struggle with the auto-immune disease lupus, she wrote to one of her friends, "Pain is a place."

Yes, I thought, pain *is* a place. And you go there by yourself. When we lie in bed alone in a hospital room, we can let the walls close in on us and experience ourselves as cut off from the human family. We can tell ourselves, "I am the only one having this experience, and no one else knows what I'm going through." And, in a way, this is true.

Intense pain sends you out all alone on a little boat in a great sea inside yourself, and it blurs the world outside your skin. The world marches right on, but what goes on outside of you takes on a strange, far-away character. You look at it all as if from a great distance and often with very little interest. Pain takes us hostage – especially our attention. Enduring intense physical pain requires our full attention simply to move from one moment to the next. I was far out at sea on my tiny boat – hanging on for dear life as the waves pounded over me, threatening to overturn my fragile craft and leave me to drown.

But from time to time I would open my eyes. And I would see – as if through a dense fog – my family and friends. It was as if they stood watch on a distant shore, keeping me from becoming completely lost. I knew that when the time came for me to return, their faithful vigil would be a beacon for the journey back. We need our people to keep the light on and the door open so that we can find our bearings and make our way back home when we're ready.

It's possible to experience pain so agonizing that it completely owns us. I can testify to enduring pain that made me totally oblivious to everything and everybody around me. After those experiences, I recall very little about where I was, who else was there, and what else was going on outside of me. I was completely inside myself, and those who cared for me had to push themselves into "my place" to reach me.

The late lawyer and lay theologian William Stringfellow, who has been a great influence on those of us at the Open Door and many other Christian disciples, spent many years grappling with physical pain and illness. He wrote that pain is an acolyte for the power of death. Even when a reprieve comes, the sufferer knows that they have experienced a foretaste of dying.

Those of us who have suffered such extended and excruciating pain wonder in the throes of it whether it will ever end – and not knowing complicates the agony. We come to recognize the desperate place within us that would do virtually *anything* to end the pain. Thankfully, each of my many episodes of such suffering came to an end. These harsh and unwelcomed experiences have forced into my consciousness and prayers those who live this day with chronic and unrelenting pain.

Illness and pain can become an opportunity for re-inhabiting our bodies. Bodies carry memory and solidarity with the creation that we often have "forgotten" or suppressed. "Re-membering" ourselves is an opportunity for deepening our incarnational theology – the stunning awareness that God chose to come to earth in the flesh and share our sufferings.

Though pain can be isolating, it can also be a bridge. When I can creep out of my own place of suffering long enough, I see the others who suffer: their faces, tired and worn from their troubles; their brave smiles and faithful thanksgivings for another day of life, for "coming this far by faith"; their confident declarations that "God hasn't brought me this far to leave me now."

My pain belongs not just to me but to the human family. It can make me think only of myself and my desire for relief – or it can become a deep cry from my own depths for the pain of all who suffer. Hospitals and clinic waiting rooms can be a very helpful geography for this journey – and for those who journey with us.

The intestinal blockage in May was the first of several that plagued me that summer of 1995, two severe enough to require hospitalization. My extensive surgery had caused adhesions – scar tissue –that crisscrossed my abdomen. They periodically caught my intestines and tied them in knots like a twisted balloon. Sometimes such blockages necessitate more surgery; and sometimes the intestines, which constantly float and shift in our abdomens, unfurl themselves, which thankfully happened for me.

But this first episode brought yet another big step into humility. To be very sick is to encounter many issues that you might have thought you could not bear for anyone to know. But if you're in the hospital, the truth is just out there, and there's nothing you can do to hide it and preserve your dignity. Friends want the facts so that they can know how to pray and help you heal. Once the path was cleared, I felt like pretty much everybody in Atlanta – and many people beyond – were praying for my bowels to wake up. "Moving" prayers were offered in many corners.

One night before the sought-for result, my wonderful, petite nurse friend Ms. Rucker was leaving my room. "Ms. Davis," she said, turning with a mischievous grin as she walked out my door, "did anybody ever tell you you're full of it?"

I laughed and told her yes. Later, I wished I had said, "Yes, but this is the first time there's been an X-ray to prove it." Or maybe, "Yes, but this is the first time it's required hospitalization."

Once things started moving again and the abdominal pressure was relieved, the NG tube came out, the awful headache went away, and I began to feel like myself again. It was then that I began to be annoyed and distracted that I had more clumps of hair on my clothes and pillow than on my head. "When you come to see me tonight," I told Hannah over the phone one day, "bring the clippers and scissors. I'm ready for The Haircut."

That evening in my hospital room, Hannah, Ed, Dot, and Marilyn Washburn, along with the nurses who came in and out, helped me conjure a party atmosphere for Hannah's work. She carefully cut chunks of my thinning locks, ran the clippers over the stubble, and then shaved what was left. I emerged with a shiny bald dome.

I began to explore the adventure of being a bald-headed woman. For most of us, our hair and our sense of self are at least somewhat tangled, shall we say. It definitely took some getting used to, and there were times when I felt a bit shy about my new "do." But sometimes I felt that my lack of hair – not to mention my pasty paleness during chemo – had more of an effect on others than on me. At times I slapped on a scarf and a swipe of lipstick just so my friends and family wouldn't worry so much.

I found over time that I could work with my baldness, and even enjoy it. Friends contributed scarves and hats, silly and serious, and Hannah and Dot and I experimented with different ways to tie and combine them. My few experiments with wigs were singularly unimpressive and uncomfortable, so I abandoned that option quickly. I learned that summer was in fact a very convenient time to be bald – especially living in Atlanta without air conditioning. I did my best to take it lightly and see the upside of hairlessness, and I was especially happy not to be trailing wisps and drifts of hair everywhere I went.

Yvonne King, a retired professor of languages who had come through a rough battle with breast cancer, quickly assembled and sent me a "Chemotherapy Survival Kit." It contained crystallized ginger to help with nausea, a sleep mask for daytime naps, and lots of comical little items to keep us laughing. Once again, I was thankful that friends and humor were available to see us through.

July's repeat performance was even more awful than May's event. I was eating mint chocolate chip ice cream with Ed and Joyce, who was back for another visit, when I was seized by a wracking pain. I managed a chuckle when Ed joked, "Joyce is back, time for another intestinal blockage." And then I disappeared into the truth of his proclamation and a world of misery.

I threw up for hours on end – in whatever bag, basin, or trash can was available – as I moved through Grady from the clinic to the Emergency Room to the Radiology wing. Sitting on the edge of a cold, steel table, I wept when a nurse handed me a large glass filled with a heavy, chalky, white liquid and told me I had to drink it. Such was the protocol for a barium-swallow X-ray. When you're vomiting green stuff and not really at your social best, it's comforting to be gently assured that barium is so heavy that, no matter how many times you throw up, it will stay put.

There in the dark recesses of Radiology, I met two of the sweetest caregivers I have encountered in my long journey with illness. "I know this is hard, darlin'," said X-ray technician Alisa Hulsey as she held a basin for me, "but keep trying."

"You're doin' fine, sweetness," chimed in radiologist Dr. Arthur Fountain, as he wiped my face with a cool, wet cloth. These two professionals attended me like ministering angels. I couldn't see past my excruciating pain, but they came across that barrier to me. Though they could not remove my suffering, they offered the comfort and reassurance that I desperately needed. I will love them forever for their empathy and kindness at a point of my deepest need.

A few days later, doctors ordered a second X-ray. I was hoping for the revelation of good news, so that I could be released from the hospital and go home. It was a quiet Sunday morning, I was feeling much better, and everything was looking like sunshine. Ed helped me into a wheelchair and covered me with a sheet. While I pulled my IV pole along, he wheeled me down the hall to the elevator and on to Radiology on the third floor. The nurses and technicians at the nurses' station greeted us warmly.

After the X-ray, Ed asked me, "Do you feel like you could walk a little bit?" and I answered "Sure." When I got out, Ed climbed quickly into the chair, wrapped the sheet around his head and shoulders, and grabbed the IV pole, looking as pathetic as he could. I pushed him out toward the nurses' station as if this were perfectly normal. The women at the station did a double-take, looking horrified.

At the time, Georgia Congressman Newt Gingrich, soon to be Speaker of the U.S. House of Representatives, was pushing a plan that would have gutted federal support of healthcare for the poor. As we passed the nurses' station, Ed yelled, "It's the Newt Gingrich healthcare plan: the sick push the healthy!" The nurses and technicians could not contain themselves, bursting into gales of laughter. They were still laughing as the door swung shut behind us.

Ed and I traded places for the trip in the elevator and then switched again when we got up to 10-A. We repeated the farce as we passed the nurses' station there, evoking the same reaction. After the laughter subsided, one of the nurses looked at Ed and said, "You have no idea how much you help us when you make us laugh."

Truth be told, it helped us all.

7

Into the Stillness

"Oh, this must be *terrible* for you," a friend said to me, "not to be able to do your work." She was one among many who offered such a sentiment of sympathy. But as curious as it seemed, I thought in response, *No. In the first place, I'm working really hard. And in the second place, I feel that although the disease is terrible, the work before me is not.*

Eventually I remembered a statement by William Stringfellow, written as he faced his life-threatening illness: "My vocation is to be William Stringfellow: nothing more, nothing less." When I had first read those words in his autobiography *Second Birthday* many years before, they seemed simplistic. But in the throes of chemotherapy in the summer of 1995, I began to understand what he meant.

My work for almost 20 years had been as a pastor and advocate with prisoners and homeless people. My work changed dramatically that summer. I was not driving back and forth to death row. I was not making soup for our Open Door soup kitchen. I was not writing letters to prisoners or articles for our newspaper, *Hospitality*. I was not preaching or leading worship, providing music or making speeches about human rights at political rallies.

If I understood my work as my vocation, then my illness was a drastic and disturbing interruption. But I came to see that though my work had changed, my vocation had not. The real question for me was: Who am I called to be in this radically changed situation of my life? My vocation was what it had always been: to be Murphy Davis – nothing more, nothing less.

I certainly had no lack of work to do. My days were a full regimen of taking medications, changing bandages, resting, going to the clinic, receiving chemo injections, resting, eating, resting, visiting with friends and family, resting, resting, resting. My work was clearly set out for me, and I was working hard. It took all my energy between spells of sleep just to put one foot in front of the other and keep going.

My "one day at a time" struggle to move toward recovery from a disease that had attacked my entire physical being deepened my appreciation for my many friends who have found hope in the discipline and patience of 12-step programs. Sometimes it was a "one minute at a time" journey for me. Walking through my illness gave me a profound understanding of what author Reynolds Price aptly called "the moment-by-moment task of healing."

In those difficult days of treatment and recovery, I found sustenance in scripture and in the unrelenting love of my family and friends. Our good friend Pete Gathje, then a university professor in Memphis, directed Ed and me to the 43rd chapter of Isaiah. The words we found there became a mainstay for my meditation and a hope for all of us at the Open Door Community during my treatment and recovery:

> *Do not be afraid – I will save you.*
> *I have called you by name – you are mine.*
> *When you pass through deep waters, I will be with you;*
> *Your troubles will not overwhelm you.*
> *When you pass through fire you will not be burned;*
> *The hard trials that come will not hurt you.*
> *For I am the Holy One,*
> *The God who saves you.* (Is. 43:1b-3a)

Living through cancer gives one a clear answer to the question, What do I know by heart? Over and over that summer, as I traipsed from one clinic to another and endured one test after another, the 23rd Psalm just sort of started up in my head. The first time I was aware of it was on the inside of a metal capsule having an MRI: *The Lord is my shepherd*...whrrrrrr...*I shall not*....bangbangbangbang...*want.* "You lead me beside still waters; you restore my soul" became an ever-present mantra of comfort.

Still waters. Oh, how I craved stillness.

I got it from time to time – mostly in the middle of the night. I began routinely waking up sometime between 3 and 6 o'clock in the morning, unable to return to sleep for one, two, three hours at a time. This interruption seemed related to my medication cycles.

The uninvited wakefulness initially angered and frustrated me: *With all that I am dealing with, can't I at least get a good night's sleep?* I resisted it and fought to return to sleep. And then I started to see these moments as a gift.

I had known instinctively early on that my drastic illness was not unrelated to my unceasing activity over the years; I had to learn that my healing must come from stillness. I wrote in my journal:

That which comes to heal us
can speak only in the
silence within us.

I began to focus again on my prayer life, which had been strong in the hospital but had become scattered and diminished at home. This was not a new reality for me. I had always struggled to slow down enough to pay attention to my inner life. My journal reflects my wrestlings:

May 12, 1995, 3:00 a.m.

Early-morning wakefulness has returned...We'll see if it will mean more journaling and meditation time. No rash promises. I continue to try not to impose an agenda on myself – with some curiosity about what "just emerges." On the other hand, I don't want to fall into an entrenched pattern of sloth and disorganization. At some point I want to be more serious about my work – soul work and the more outward sort...

But can I be about what has been my work once again without pushing myself into a mode or posture of illness? Have I made myself sick? Did I earn this cancer with a frantic lifestyle? Did the aggressive tumors take over in the depth of my woman-ness and my bowels for lack of attentiveness and care – for lack of nourishment and soul work? For lack of oxygen and sunshine?

Or does it matter at all?

I am not anxious. I have been vigilant about not charging myself guilty of causing my lymphoma. There are many things I could point to over the years that have been problems in my lifestyle: lack of exercise, lack of attentiveness at many points to diet and, especially, stress – high-level, intense, fatiguing, overwhelming, and sometimes unrelenting stress. And chronic fatigue. I have been very hard on my body and my soul.

I do not regret the life I have lived to this point. I am deeply grateful for all that I have been able to know and have and do. But it has been hard.

I am in a fight for my life. I want with all my heart, mind, soul, and spirit to be healed. My cancer is very aggressive and fast-growing. But it is no match for the combination of mega-chemotherapy and prayers of supplication and intercession coming from literally around the world. No match.

My hope and prayer is that the tumors don't stand a chance.

The night after writing this, I had a very memorable dream, which unfolded like this: I am at a conference in a Southern plantation house. Many things are going on at once, and I am apparently responsible for all the arrangements. The childcare worker comes only intermittently. She gets all the babies and small children to have a crawling race, and they're going everywhere, in all directions. I pick up a baby with a loaded, overflowing diaper. But I'm supposed to be at a meeting with civil rights leaders. I've missed the meeting, and therefore also an important connection to help prisoners and impoverished people in Georgia, an angry and disappointed group of whom show up looking for me.

I wrote the following reflection in my journal the next morning:

I seem to be grappling with lots of responsibility residue. How will things go on without me? How will the needy people I serve get by? How will I get by without being constantly in charge and responsible? (Aha! Perhaps the key question!)

Can I let it go? I hope in the future to lower the compulsion level of my responsibility syndrome. That task is on me now – learning to let go, to trust, to allow things to flow.

I wrote, "I am a compulsive connector. It is perhaps my best gift – and it has become a burden, if not a curse." Hospitality and networking were part of my family heritage, and I had cultivated them into a fine art by the time I was a young adult. How amazing that I received a hundred pieces of mail every week after my surgery that summer from friends, colleagues, supporters, and allies across the country and around the world – not to mention a deluge of flowers, gifts, visits, and calls. This truth overwhelmed me with gratitude and joy. But I wanted to be able to trust this connectedness, to enjoy it and let it be. I longed to be able to nurture and tend these relationships without working so frantically and compulsively at them.

I began paying closer attention to my dreams, knowing that they are messages from the soul about its desires, its ruminations, its attachments – one of the very important ways God's Spirit whispers to us. The images became more vivid and troubling: I'm late to the airport for a flight to a speaking engagement and speeding in the car, but I can't find the exit ramp. A friend of Hannah's is pregnant and wants me to preside at the wedding for her and her boyfriend, who I think is drinking and abusing her. I'm an FBI agent/spy dressed in a trench coat and Dick Tracy fedora, standing ramrod straight next to a young child in a closet, where I get discovered and sent on a high-risk assignment.

In an especially detailed dream, I want to take my pretty nightgown with matching robe to the hospital, but my mother is wearing it as a dress and doesn't want to give it up, so I fume at her. Down the hall I find that my rocking chair has been broken, and I am furious. Ed has replaced the doors in our apartment with aluminum storm doors that are tacky and ugly, and I yell at him. I go into the bathroom, and it immediately fills up with visitors, college students who won't leave me alone. I scream at them, too: "This is *my* bathroom. You are *not* invited here. You are *not* welcome here. Get out. NOW!"

Not exactly subtly, my dreams were trying to help me get the messages I needed to hear about responsibility, anxiety, boundaries, limitations, and letting go. On May 22nd, I wrote just two sentences in my journal: "The tumors grew fastest in my mothering organs. Is this an indication of an over-extended or stressed mothering impulse or vocation in me?"

After my initial surgery, which included a hysterectomy, I emerged "older and wiser," in some sense, feeling that I had sent my younger self off to the incinerator with all my obsolete organs. I had lost my generative, "creative" organs and wondered what this would mean as I was shoved into a different phase of life. I was trying desperately to "lay to rest" my old self and embrace this "new creation" that was me. That task was – and still is – my most challenging one. I have known from the very beginning that this was a critical part of my healing, but I have shrunk from it again and again.

My dear friend Nelia Kimbrough sent me some guided-imagery tapes by Belleruth Naperstek. The most memorable section included these lines: "I tell my cancer these things: Thank you for teaching me to stop and listen. Thank you for reminding me of what is truly important. You can go now." I repeated that command "You can go now" like a mantra. Naperstek continued: "I know that I have things to do, gifts to give, purposes to accomplish. I require a healthy working body for this."

Friends sent Ed and me letters, articles, and books to help us along in understanding the illness that was wracking my body and in navigating its challenges to our soul journey. Yvonne and Allen King gave us Michael Leunig's lovely little book *The Prayer Tree*. One of the prayers became a constant companion for us:

Dear God,
We pray for another way of being: another way of knowing.
Across the difficult terrain of our existence we have attempted to build a highway and in so doing have lost our footpath.
God, lead us to our footpath: Lead us there where in simplicity we may move at the speed of natural creatures and feel the earth's love beneath our feet.
Lead us there where step-by-step we may feel the movement of creation in our hearts. And lead us there where side-by-side we may feel the embrace of the common soul.
Nothing can be loved at speed. God lead us to the slow path; to the joyous insights of the pilgrim; another way of knowing: another way of being. Amen.

Nothing can be loved at speed. Indeed! For some years Ed had been repeating this motto: "Truth only moves at three miles an hour." That, he explained, is because three miles per hour is about the speed that a human being can move by foot – or on a donkey. To live life at any depth, speed has to go.

This is a formidable challenge in our era. Relentless activity at a frenetic pace is the norm in our culture. We rush from one obligation or task to another, living by schedules and calendars – rarely staying "in the moment" to be present to what is going on, or to those with whom we share the moment, or even to ourselves. My cancer had enforced a reduced speed, but I was already beginning to wonder how I would carry this speed limit into the future.

My cousin Carol Williams sent me a copy of Kat Duff's *The Alchemy of Illness*. It "spoke to my condition," as they say. Duff's descriptions of the "work" of illness helped me to put words to the labor that was so different from anything I had ever done before: those "long hours in bed suspended between worlds," taking me "over and over the tangled lines of my life." She speaks of apologies unmade and gratitude unspoken, of gardens untended and dreams denied. She acknowledges that many things can't be undone. But, she wrote, "I can pay attention…to remember, to mourn, and honor, to clear myself of these entangling lines while holding the entire snarl as sacred."

This is, according to Duff, "tedious, tenuous, and lifegiving labor," in which there is no role for "grand heroic gestures." It involves patience, small steps, and few words, treating ourselves with "the tenderness of baby-catching hands, remembering that we find our power, our capacity to heal ourselves and our world, in our deep and abiding vulnerability."

The heart of the great labor of illness, says Duff, is *listening*: attending carefully to the particulars of one's own experience. I knew what I had been listening *to*: my body, my dreams, all that I needed to know about this disease and how I could heal from it, body and spirit. But I found Kat Duff a helpful guide in discerning what I was listening *for*. She wrote that one of the requirements of healing is to "reclaim one's soul – that vital essence that enables us to thrive – and resume one's 'path of destiny.'" This task includes, according to Duff, calling up and re-inhabiting our lost memories, listening to our dreams and intuitions, and being honest with ourselves and others about our true feelings and desires. "Soul retrieval" is work. Our bodies bear memories that our minds have ignored or forgotten, and it takes time to listen as they find space to come to consciousness.

In "Afterthoughts," a conversation that writer-activist Marge Piercy had with Ira Wood around 2014, she said she "treated my body as a renewable resource." She slept little and pushed a lot, believing her energy to be inexhaustible. But to do so is to live beyond the boundaries that are established for human life. Duff uses the image of a life savings of energy. When it is used up, all that is left is a "checking account," which will be drawn down to zero if it is not replenished.

According to Duff, hubris – the human desire to push our limits and feel powerful, to go "beyond the allotted portion" – is "slain in illness to nurture reverence and humility – human littleness in relation to a greater Mystery." Spirit as well as body must have rest: time to cogitate and ruminate, to remember and recall, to hold in perspective both human belovedness and smallness.

And the human spirit cannot live at speed. When we rush through life, our spirits cannot keep up. Illness forces us to stop. If we do not take the opportunity to listen, to gently and patiently reach back to retrieve some of what has been left behind, then we cannot heal. We cannot take up our lives to move forward with a deeper wisdom. We are not responsible *for* our illnesses, wrote Duff, we are responsible *to* them – to what they offer and require of us.

Thankfully, miraculously, against all odds, the chemo and prayers did their work. My chemotherapy treatment was completed at the end of August. But recovery is a slow and gradual process. Although I would not have wanted to be anywhere else, and the questions would have plagued me anywhere, the Open Door Community, like modern life generally, was a difficult place to be "in between." The issues that had begun to surface when I entered treatment felt relentless: How do I work and rest in a healthy cycle? How do I limit stress? How do I find boundaries in the face of endless need and demand? How can I be in true solidarity with those in need without getting overwhelmed by their suffering – or my own?

It became very clear to me why Kat Duff pointed to the serious dilemma of this period. The great temptation is to "re-cover": to cover over the time of illness, to forget about it and rush on as if it had never happened. But the need for the footpath – the slow pace that allows for remembrance and meditation and time to honor the wisdom revealed in a serious illness – remained.

This was really the hard part. When you've been ill, most people want you to "get back to normal" as quickly as possible. The needs that waited patiently during the illness begin clamoring for attention. How to go forward without falling back into the frenetic pace?

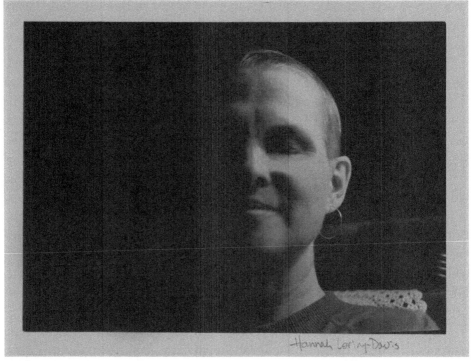

"Out of the Shadow,"by Hannah Loring-Davis, made for a photography class she took in the fall of 1995 with George Mitchell - a great depiction of Murphy's movement from treatment and the shadow of cancer back into "normal" life.

I would never say that I was happy to have had such a close brush with death. But there is no denying that many blessings have come to me that I would otherwise never have experienced. One of those is the hard reminder that without focused quiet reflection and prayer, we run the risk of becoming fragile, brittle, shallow, soul-less people.

I had known this truth before my illness, but I had neglected the importance of it. In the frantic years of activism, resistance, and hospitality work, the needs were just so great that I could always justify to myself rushing on and neglecting the time for pondering and meditation. Now I realized that the path of least resistance would be to plow back into a full schedule. That would reassure a lot of people. It would help us all to forget that this unpleasant period of my life had ever happened.

While I did not suffer the illusion that I had "caused" my own illness, I knew, as Kat Duff reminded me, that I had to be responsible to what I had experienced and learned. And part of that meant living at a pace that was more in tune with the needs of my body and soul. The many changes that my body had gone through had to be honored in some way, and the needs of my spirit and soul required my continuing attention.

God's Spirit rarely shouts from deep inside of us. In our day-to-day lives, the voice of the Spirit within us usually speaks in whispers. We do not hear this "still small voice" readily when we are rushing around. So if we act and live only out of will and obligation, we miss the depth of life that comes when we are quiet and still enough to hear the important messages of our inner life. Our dreams often speak to us of the desires of our soul, but the messages are often lost with the morning light because we do not take the time to listen.

In the summer of 1995, this was – and it will continue to be for the rest of my life – a serious dilemma. *How are we to live in solidarity with the suffering and dying poor of the earth without working in a way that is so frantic that it renders our physical and mental health vulnerable to disease and disorders?* This is not just my personal issue; it is one that haunts most of us in the activist community. With the notable exception of the many people who are unemployed or in prison, the dilemma of frantic activity is a plague in our techno-industrial society, and those of us who work for something other than money and endless consumption are not exempt.

Grace frequently comes in strange and unanticipated forms and expressions. And however it comes, we often resist it. Receiving grace and making the changes that grace might require demand concentration and discipline. Change doesn't "just happen." It is labor.

The establishment of new regimens of lifestyle, the physical disciplines to enhance the immune system and take responsibility for one's own health, the structured time for soul work – all of this requires focused effort. It is not something you just "tack on" to an already busy routine. It is an unending learning process and effort. All I have learned to do with it is to befriend the tension and do the best I can in its presence.

One day in November 1995, three months after the end of my chemotherapy, Ed and I were sharing lunch, discussing something routine and unmemorable, when I suddenly burst into tears. This rush of emotion, seeming to come out of nowhere, startled me. I knew immediately that my illness had something yet to teach me.

I began to take stock of the fact that, for all the anxiety and physical suffering of my cancer journey, it had contained quite a sweetness. Never, ever, had I imagined such a time of being completely surrounded and held tight by the love, care, and concern of hundreds of family members and friends far and near. It was all quite overwhelming. And then it was over. Once my treatments were finished, gone were the frequent trips to Grady and the conversations and attention from my doctors and nurses there. Visits from friends tapered off. Flowers and gifts stopped arriving. I had to catch myself and ask, Am I wishing I could be sick again?

Not hardly, as they say. But, in the midst of my overwhelming gratitude and joy at having been given back my life, I also experienced a letdown. Something was definitely gone from my daily existence that I was missing. A sweet intensity. A slow pace. Stillness. Time to reflect and talk quietly. Living in the present – one day at a time.

Months before, when I was in the throes of trying to find an answer to my mysterious ailments and finally getting on a clear path toward diagnosis, my mother had sent me a letter that offered her wisdom and insight on this truth about my life:

So glad that answers are coming on your epizootics! How thankful we are that things are definitely looking up. Now – this is your mother speaking – work on pacing yourself! If you don't look after it, no one will. You and Ed are too valuable to society and the kingdom of God, to your family and friends, to fail to take care of yourselves. Old age brings on many health problems, and no use bringing them on earlier than you have to! Pop and I have been in good health for so long, just realize that we've been blessed, and old age is slower catching up on us. You don't want to get old before your time!

She was right, of course, about pacing myself. A mother knows her daughter as no one else can. Ironically, Mama died of pancreatic cancer at the age of 85 two years later, on February 15, 1997. She was herself to the very end: loving, honest, fun, grateful, faith-filled. She organized a sort of Dying Party at the Presbyterian Home in High Point, North Carolina, where she and my Dad lived.

In the infirmary, as the end was nearing, family and friends were coming by to gather around her bed, along with a few younger friends to whom she had been like a mother, including Sally and her husband, Don. Mama's voice was very weak, and she was being more quiet than usual. But she rallied enough to pick up a spoon and bang it on the railing of the hospital bed. When she had everyone's attention, she said quietly, "I want to thank you for being such wonderful friends. The only regret I have is...Don, I'm gonna die, and you're still a Republican!"

That was a hard year. Though the grief I felt was greatest for my mother, I also lost 12 other family members and friends I was close to in 1997. I accompanied some of them, including Patsy Morris and Kathleen Carlin, on their journeys with chemotherapy and cancer, offering what wisdom I could about rest and self-care, hope and head coverings. With each death, I felt caught in a paradox: feeling great gratitude for all the lives that have deeply touched mine – and facing the challenge of how to honor all these wonderful connections without being overwhelmed by them.

That was also the year that Hannah graduated from high school. What rejoicing that I had lived to see that day! And then the hard truth hit that it was time to let her go as well. It was not a permanent release, of course, and I knew that Hannah would always be very much a part of my life. But watching her go off to college that fall was bittersweet, deepening the sense of emptiness that gnawed at me and threatened to take up residence in my heart.

8

Taking Politics Personally

It was a hot morning in downtown Decatur, on the eastern edge of Atlanta. Police were swarming the streets around the County Administration Building where the DeKalb County commissioners were about to meet. Jail buses were lined up in the parking lot. Both state and local police sharpshooters were poised and ready on top of surrounding buildings and parking decks.

We were certainly not new to activism. Over the years, those of us from the Open Door Community frequently could be found on the streets, or in local political offices, regularly advocating for the needs of Atlanta's poorest citizens. We had marched for affordable housing and against the death penalty. We were engaged in longtime resistance to the city's attempts to enforce a "vagrant-free zone," which included rounding up people from the streets for loitering or public urination – stepped up dramatically when the Olympics came to Atlanta in the summer of 1996. We advocated for public toilets in the downtown area, holding protests in Woodruff Park and hauling a toilet into the mayor's office to make a point.

Most business leaders and city officials vehemently opposed our efforts, arguing that meeting the needs of its poor citizens would make Atlanta a "magnet" for homeless persons. We did, however, have one stunning success, well documented in *Raising Our Voices, Breaking the Chain*, written by our friend Terry Easton. For two weeks in June 1990, we had occupied the massive, abandoned Imperial Hotel on Peachtree Street. Once an SRO (single resident occupancy) hotel providing low-cost housing, it had been purchased and closed down by a wealthy developer with big, upscale plans that hadn't materialized.

We demanded that it once again house poor people, more than 300 of whom came in off the streets and joined us in the occupation.

Through a long and complicated process over more than six years after our occupation, with continuing pressure and the partnership of developer Bruce Gunter, The Imperial reopened on December 18, 1996. It contained 120 low-income apartments and on-site support services for tenants with physical disabilities, addiction problems, mental health issues, and employment needs.

Among its first tenants was Karen Thomas, one of several people needing housing that my friend Albertine Yorke had sent our way from Grady Hospital. It got to be a joke between my social worker and me that, whenever I was getting ready to leave the hospital she would ask, "How many people are you going to take home this time?"

Karen Thomas had suffered from childhood encephalitis, and she walked with an elevated shoe and the aid of a wrap-around metal crutch. Though they would have been hers for the asking, she never claimed her right to Medicaid and Disability payments. Instead, she worked for 20 years at a desk job with the Atlanta Police Department, until she developed breast cancer. When she had surgery and started chemotherapy for the cancer, Karen lost her job. Along with her job, she lost her health insurance.

I learned "up close and personal" for the first time what it meant to have employment-based health care. Karen Thomas had paid into her health care plan for 20 years. But when she got sick and needed it, she lost the job *and the insurance* after just a few months of treatment. She had run out of rent money and was one day away from homelessness when she came to live with us. Thank God for my social worker, Ms. Yorke, who sent her to us! Karen was a wonderful addition to the Open Door, staying with us for about a year while she went through chemotherapy, until she took up residence in The Imperial. Sadly, she lived only two months there before the cancer claimed her life.

During the Imperial Hotel occupation, as with all our campaigns involving civil disobedience, we were generously served by our wonderful friend Brian Spears, a lawyer who contributed countless pro bono hours to us over the years. He had also helped Ed and me get our living wills and power-of-attorney documents together when the doctors told us to "get our affairs in order." His partner Ellen Spears, a renowned environmental historian, and their marvelous children Lelia and Ben, then teenagers, were mainstays of friendship and strong supporters of our street actions from our earliest years in Atlanta.

So, yes, we were used to making a ruckus on behalf of justice. But even those of us with decades of protest activity behind us were a bit stunned by this display of force in Decatur. It was May of 1999, and the lives of Grady patients and the future of the hospital were on the line. Never had a political campaign felt so personal to me. I had learned in the women's movement of the 1960s and '70s that "the political is personal, and the personal is political." That felt true to my experience more than ever.

Grady Hospital had saved my life. If I had been living in an underserved rural area – or a city such as Milwaukee or Washington, D.C., which had already dismantled their "safety net" hospitals – I would probably have died. At the time, an estimated 20,000 people were dying every year in the U.S. because they lacked health insurance and couldn't get the care they needed.

After the completion of my chemo in the summer of 1995, I had relied on Grady for follow-up clinic visits and a CAT scan every three months. Burkitt's lymphoma is very likely to recur, and when it does, it's usually within two to three years. I needed those follow-up visits and scans to monitor my health and catch any changes.

In the fall of 1997, a routine scan had revealed something suspicious in my abdomen, and the doctors ordered a biopsy. Expecting to get the results in three to five days, I was rolled into the scanner lying on my belly with an anesthetized lower back. Ed joined the doctors and technicians behind a pane of glass, one of whom operated the needle to biopsy the suspicious node.

Suddenly I heard a commotion erupt among them. *What in the world?* Face down inside the big scanner, I couldn't exactly turn around to see what was going on. But the hum of the moving table let me know I would soon rejoin them. They were practically jumping for joy. "It's a vein!" somebody shouted. "It's just a *vein!*" I had no idea what they were talking about, and my foggy brain could not fathom why they were so jubilant.

"The needle just drew blood," came the explanation. "It's not a node at all."

Wow. I did not have a recurrence of cancer. I had a varicose vein in my abdomen. Hallelujah.

In January 1998, I saw Dr. Sam Newcom for my regular clinic visit. He walked briskly into the examining room – all smiles – and slapped my chart on the table. "I don't know why we don't just call you *cured!*"

Cured? Did he actually use that word? Is it possible? Once again, I remembered the death sentence I had been given two and a half years before: six to 18 months to live. I looked at him and wondered, Are you talking to *me?*

He *was* talking to me. "We're calling this a cure," he repeated.

Dr. Newcom reminded us once again that Burkitt cells double in size every 30 days. He explained that, unlike some other cancers, Burkitt cells cannot be present without growing. If they haven't shown up again within three years, the prognosis is that they aren't going to.

If Dr. Newcom said I was cured, I knew for sure that I was cured. What I didn't know was that that clinic visit would be my last with him.

My 50th birthday arrived two months later. My family and community decided that this was a birthday that needed to be celebrated *big*. A throng gathered in the basement of Druid Hills Presbyterian Church for a feast and party. Our friend Craig Rafuse pulled together a rock-and-roll band that played for everybody to dance. Many stories were told, and guests were particularly amused to hear about the many silly things I had said and done while under the influence of pain medication. Among those who attended were Dr. Newcom and his wife, Janis, and my nurses Nancy Feldman and Rick White and their partners. For somebody who wasn't supposed to see a 48th birthday, turning 50 was *sweet*.

When I returned to Grady for my next clinic visit, Dr. Newcom was not there. I saw another hematologist, one I had never met before. As I checked out, I asked the nurse coordinator about Dr. Newcom. She said simply, "Dr. Newcom is no longer with Grady or Emory." That was it. No other details were offered. It seemed very curious, because Dr. Newcom was deeply committed to the hospital and to his Grady patients.

I later heard that he had been fired. That seemed impossible to believe. Then I saw a letter to the editor in the *Atlanta Journal Constitution* from Dr. Newcom himself. He was protesting a new co-pay policy that had been passed by the Fulton-DeKalb Hospital Authority, which oversaw the administration of Grady.

The hospital board had voted to impose a mandatory co-pay of 10 dollars per prescription and five dollars per clinic visit, effective March 1, 1999. For AIDS patients who depended on as many as 30 medications every month to keep them alive, and for the "poorest of the poor" that had been determined by Grady's own system of investigation to have zero disposable income, this represented a certain death sentence.

We learned later that a study by the hospital administration's own consultants had determined that as many as 6,500 Grady patients would die or experience "severe harm" within the first 60 days of the enforcement of this policy. The administration, including the head of the pharmacy, did not divulge these findings and recommended that the board approve the policy to enforce the co-pay.

Nothing about the question of whether or not to defend Grady was abstract or theoretical for us. For years Ed had informally monitored the Grady pharmacy and its four- to 10-hour waits for prescriptions to be filled. On just about any day of the week, you could go by there in the late morning or early afternoon and find the line stretching all the way up the hill toward Butler Street.

The excruciatingly long wait was one more of the unnecessarily punitive structures that we so often impose on the poor. If you are poor, you wait...and wait...and wait. You might have a broken foot, but you stand on it. You might be 90 years old, and you're sick and tired of being sick and tired, but you wait. You might be a weary mother with two small children, spending exasperating hours trying to corral them and calm their frantic cries. You might be a paranoid schizophrenic and begin to think there is somebody out there wanting to make your life miserable. Or you might be perfectly sane and think the same thing.

Ed's quick response to the news of the policy change was to plan a protest campaign, to begin on Monday, March 15th, the first day of the enforced co-pay. A crowd assembled on Butler Street in front of the hospital with protest signs. On that very first day of the campaign we were joined by several physicians, members of Concerned Black Clergy, many community organizers and activists, AIDS patients, and a large number of elderly Grady patients – many of them gathered from the senior-citizen centers of FACAA (Fulton Atlanta Community Action Authority).

I had called Sam Newcom at his home half an hour before we had left the Open Door for Butler Street. I explained what we were getting ready to do and said, "After I saw your letter to the editor, I just thought you might want to know."

Sam didn't hesitate. "What time will you be there?"

"Noon," I replied.

"Janis and I will see you there." I was astonished. But sure enough, when we arrived, Sam and Janis were already standing on the corner of Butler and Armstrong Streets. Sam was dressed as we had always seen him, in his immaculate, starched, long white coat, sporting his Grady name tag, with his stethoscope and percussion hammer in his pockets.

He was clearly ready for this struggle. He took the bullhorn and spoke forcefully, condemning this latest assault on Grady patients. He confirmed that patients were sure to die because of the new co-pay policy. Sam and Janis stood with us that first day, and as the Grady Campaign grew, they never missed a march, board meeting, trip to the County Commission, Grady Coalition meeting, or even the court hearings that took place after some of us were arrested.

As the weeks unfolded, we learned the story of what had happened between Dr. Newcom and Emory University School of Medicine. In 1984, the year that Dr. Newcom joined the faculty, the president of Emory University and the commissioners of Atlanta's Fulton and DeKalb Counties signed 30-year legal contracts to guarantee care for Grady patients and supplement the hospital's budget as needed.

In the early 1990s, Emory University – with an $8 billion endowment that was the sixth largest in the nation – announced several new projects. These included construction of the Winship Cancer Institute, with a $125 million price tag, and a major addition to Crawford Long Hospital, to be renamed Emory Midtown, at a cost of $275 million. Other efforts were planned: a new nursing school, suburban clinics and research buildings. Major campus alterations included a plan that was, thankfully, eventually abandoned: reconfiguring Emory University's quadrangle into the shape of a Coke bottle – in honor of the massive profits that had been funneled into the university from the lucrative Coca-Cola Corporation. (No, I'm not making this up!)

As millions of dollars poured into these other projects, Grady Hospital was being asked to bear the brunt of reductions in funding.

In 1994 Emory School of Medicine entered into a partnership with Columbia/Hospital Corporation of America, turning over clinical administrative decisions to the for-profit healthcare corporation. Its executives immediately began to explore how to cut costs. Although half of the medical school's students and faculty were at Grady at any given time, the new administrators chose Grady for cutbacks in costs and care, closing several patient programs, including the Minority Patient Cancer Program.

For a decade, Sam Newcom had been chief of Grady's Hematology Clinic and a full-time attending physician at Grady in medical oncology. He was pulled from Grady and reassigned as chief of hematology/oncology for the Veterans Administration (VA) Hospital adjacent to the Emory campus. Both of his colleagues were also reassigned, leaving Grady without a medical oncologist. Only after persistently lobbying the administrators was Dr. Newcom allowed to keep his busy weekly Hematology Clinic at Grady on Tuesdays.

Further devastation occurred in the spring of 1997, when the medical administrators proposed pulling more staff from Grady to cover private practices at the Emory Clinic and decreasing the presence of medical residents at Grady to half-time. A research fellow was purloined from the VA to help cover practices at Emory University Hospital and Emory Midtown. Emory University applied for and received $1 million from Georgia's Indigent Care Trust Fund – which, it was later revealed, was spent on student campus activities.

The medical administrators offered Dr. Newcom a promotion to full-time professor and VA employee. "The evolution of American healthcare funding has left many physicians with a terrible conflict," Dr. Newcom wrote in an article published in *Ethics & Behavior* and reprinted on the front page of our May 2000 issue of *Hospitality*. According to Dr. Newcom, William Chace, then president of Emory University, had written that physicians "are no longer bound by the Hippocratic Oath...[but] are employees under the direction of non-physician employers and therefore function under the direction of their supervisors, regardless of the best interests of their patients."

This presented Dr. Newcom with a serious ethical dilemma. According to his article, he had to ask himself, "Should I ignore the misuse of VA fellows and the severe negligence at Grady? Could I overlook the withdrawal of care from the poor and its transfer to the insured in return for a steadily rising, secure, federal salary, comfortable benefits, and a faculty promotion?"

He described unnecessarily tragic situations at the hospitals he served. A Morehouse College student had been hospitalized at Grady with leukemia. Though his sister was a perfect match for a bone marrow donation, he was denied a transplant at Emory Clinic because his father's insurance would pay only $10,000 toward it. "At the time, he was 21," wrote Dr. Newcom. "He is now dead."

An Atlanta caterer died at Grady after being given overly high doses of chemotherapy, and a Georgia Tech student died for lack of an experienced physician who could help him. A patient at the VA Hospital succumbed to a brain hemorrhage when his platelet support was arbitrarily stopped after 10 days when he reached the $2,500 limit imposed by administrators. Two others died of infections when they did not receive their immunoglobulin, which was temporarily considered too expensive for VA patients.

"I felt that I was being asked to defraud sick people and, as a teacher, to defraud physicians-in-training," wrote Dr. Newcom. "I refused to tell medical students that withholding medicine from their patients was an appropriate action or that it was necessary to accept this rationing of care. The United States was wealthy beyond all measure, and denying health care to uninsured military veterans and the poor was unacceptable to me."

Dr. Newcom went through the appropriate academic channels to register his protest. He set up meetings with Emory University officials and attempted to talk with the president who, according to Dr. Newcom, refused to meet with him. In a letter, he reminded President Chace that "the withdrawal of medical care from the VA and Grady was designed to maintain huge salaries at the Emory Clinic, some greater than $1 million to $2 million." He accused the medical administrators of "racism, greed, and reprehensible concepts of class cleansing."

Dr. Newcom was formally reprimanded. In September 1997 he was fired as chief of hematology/oncology at Grady, and the locks were changed on his office and laboratory. In April 1998 he was terminated completely at the VA. He was escorted in handcuffs to his car by three armed federal marshals. He was charged with "making written allegations of wrongdoing…that are injurious to both Emory University and to patient care." The latter was explained by saying that Dr. Newcom knew that he would be fired and was therefore denying his patients his services!

Sam Newcom sued Emory University, and the case was settled out of court. He continues to work in Atlanta as a hematology consultant. The administrators who made the decisions about staffing are no longer at Emory University School of Medicine, but the effects of their decisions remain.

It was not until I heard Sam's story that I began to understand some of my own experiences as a Grady patient. I realized then that I had never been under the care of a hematologist or oncologist when I was in the hospital. I was always treated by a rotating team of internal-medicine doctors. I saw cancer specialists only when I went to the Tuesday outpatient clinic. A year earlier, before the oncologists had been pulled from Grady, I would have received their care in the hospital.

Smiling and holding a sign proclaiming "Medicine for the Poor" at our first protest outside Grady, Sam Newcom appeared proudly in a picture on page 5 of our *Hospitality* issue that carried his article. He had done his university studies at Berkeley in California during the protest-heavy 1960s, and he had helped 25,000 marchers, including several of us from the Open Door, take back Forsyth County, Georgia, from the Ku Klux Klan in 1985. But he had never before stood in such a protest line – an experience he described as "exhilarating and empowering."

The Grady Campaign became a long and wonderful adventure. Our already diverse coalition grew to include medical students, labor union members, and some local politicians. We strategized once a week in the basement at First Iconium Baptist Church, where Ed and I often worshiped. Every time I was in the hospital, the church's "Prayer Posse" had visited me, surrounding my bed with songs and prayers and words of encouragement. The pastor, our long-time friend and co-conspirator Rev. Timothy McDonald – or Rev. Mac, as we called him – always anointed my forehead on those visits, a tangible experience of the healing power of the Spirit of Love. Rev. Mac joined Ed to co-lead the Grady coalition. We started every meeting with prayer and civil rights songs, and the spirit was solid and joyful.

We decided to take our protest directly to Edward Renford, who was hired as Grady's CEO after the public hospital he had administered in the Watts area of Los Angeles closed its doors under his leadership. A large group of us walked one day from the protest line and entered the hospital, where we were stopped on the first floor by Grady security personnel. They put Ed and Rev. Mac in handcuffs and led them away. The rest of us held our ground.

Soon one of the security officers returned and announced to us that "Rev. Loring and Rev. McDonald have asked me to tell you that everything is okay and you should disperse." *How stupid did he think we were?*

Rev. Fred Taylor, a renowned civil rights advocate and long-time staff member with SCLC (Southern Christian Leadership Conference), stepped up and declared, "We are sure that you are a nice man. But we do not operate that way. Reverends McDonald and Loring would surely not communicate with us through you." We stayed put.

Reverends Mac and Ed eventually returned. Hospital personnel informed us that Mr. Renford was away from the hospital at a Rotary meeting. We still stayed put. Finally Renford – who had been there all along – relented, and we were ushered into his executive suite. We had a conversation that, amazingly, lasted five-and-a-half hours. He ended it by promising us that no patient would leave Grady without needed medication and signed a statement to that effect.

But Dr. Neil Shulman, a hypertension specialist and Emory faculty member, began documenting that patients were still being forced from the pharmacy without medication. One of these was Ron Spencer, a homeless man who had suffered a stroke and came to live with us at the Open Door.

We decided to take our protest to the Fulton-DeKalb Hospital Authority, to demand that the board rescind, or at least temporarily suspend, its decision to impose the co-pay for prescriptions and clinic visits. Every day the policy was in place was a threat to the lives and wellbeing of Grady patients. On March 22nd, we went en masse to a meeting of the board, filling all the available seats and standing crammed along the walls. Ron sat in his wheelchair, moaning from pain. He begged the board to give him relief. Others of us spoke about the death-dealing nature of the new policy.

Despite our pleas, the board voted to leave the odious policy in place. The room exploded. We jumped to our feet and began to cry out in protest and then chant in unison: "Medicine for the poor," and "Shame on the board," and "We shall not be moved." With looks of utter terror on their faces, the board members fled the room, quickly locking the door behind them.

Security personnel began to push us around and demand order. After things quieted down a bit, the board members filed back into the room and returned to their places. They took another vote and suspended the policy for 30 days. At a subsequent meeting, it was permanently shelved.

After the vote, one of the board members lectured us about Grady's serious financial trouble and told us we should help them raise the money needed for the hospital to survive. From our very first meetings, we had tried to make clear to the administrators and members of the board that we wanted to work in partnership with them. Though it was astounding to us that they remained so passive in the face of massive cuts from federal, state, and local governments, we took their plea seriously.

So our next task was to advocate that the Fulton and DeKalb County governments pay their financial obligations to the hospital, based on the 30-year contracts they had signed. Our large and loud group appeared at a meeting of the Fulton County Commission, chanting for justice. The commission chair, a large white man who was retired from a career in professional football with the Atlanta Falcons, demanded that we take our seats and be quiet. When our diverse and energized group stood firm, he threatened to call the police.

We got louder. The commissioners agreed to grant us a full hearing on the subject of their financial obligation to Grady. When we finished speaking, the majority of the commission members voted to send the $3.5 million they owed. They were legally obligated to pay it, but I believe we helped them overcome their delay and do the right thing.

The next site of our protest was the DeKalb County Commission, which owed Grady $1.1 million. They were a greater challenge. Reverends Mac and Ed, our most boisterous leaders, were arrested during our first attempt to meet with the commission. Officer M.D. Jones of the DeKalb County Police cursed Ed as he turned his left wrist backward, aggravating an old football injury and causing Ed pain for six weeks. While frisking Rev. Mac, another officer smashed his face against the window of the police cruiser that took them away. The office of then Atlanta Mayor Bill Campbell intervened to secure their release.

In endless meetings with members of the commission over a period of many weeks, our attempts at negotiation came to naught. Grady was facing an emergency. We felt we had to escalate our efforts. The commissioners and police apparently felt they had to escalate theirs as well. Thus we encountered downtown Decatur looking like a city under siege on May 11, 1999.

Once the commission meeting started, Rev. MacDonald rose to ask DeKalb County CEO Liane Levetan to put the needs of Grady Hospital on the agenda, as we had continually asked in the preceding weeks. She refused. Thirty of us went to the front of the auditorium, knelt in prayer, and began to sing. One by one we were raised to our feet by county police officers, handcuffed, and led out of the building to a waiting bus bound for the DeKalb County Jail.

To the best of my knowledge, this was the most diverse action of nonviolent civil disobedience in the Atlanta area since the civil rights era. We were women and men, gay and straight, Black, white, and Asian. Our group included young students and a retired Presbyterian missionary, two Buddhist nuns and an elderly Jewish labor organizer, Christian clergy, medical professionals, and members of the plumbers' and electricians' and bus drivers' unions. It was a "last hurrah" for retired labor organizer Joe Criscuolo, whose wife Goldie got arrested with us at age 83 in her dress and pumps carrying her white patent leather purse.

Two hundred supporters cheered and sang while we were loaded onto the bus. At the jail, we were welcomed by the sheriff, who was a strong supporter of our action. We were charged with disorderly conduct, and most of the protesters were released quickly.

In the nonviolent tradition of Dr. Martin Luther King, our friends Peggy Dobbins, Walter Baldwin, Douglas Dean, and Stuart Acuff, along with Ed and I, refused bail and stayed overnight. The men were kept together and shared an intense night of conversation, Bible study, and storytelling. Peggy and I were separated in the women's medical section. My mattress was like a donut, with a large hole – not just an indentation but an actual hole – in its middle. Sleep was impossible, so I spent the night reading my pocket New Testament.

The next morning we were released, ushered down to the staff cafeteria, and treated to breakfast by the sheriff. The hot grits, bacon, eggs, and biscuits were a stark contrast to the cold, hardened slop that had been served to us in the jail at 4:30 a.m. – likely a puddle of grits from the-day-before-yesterday mixed up with powered eggs.

When our group gathered on Memorial Drive in front of the jail for a press conference, Rev. Benford Stellmacher greeted us. A persistent advocate for the poor, he had heard about our witness on the radio and spent the night vigiling there with a candle and a sign that read "Letting the Light Shine for Grady Hospital." We heard the repeated honking of a city bus horn. We looked over to see Joel, a bus driver who had taken the previous day off to be arrested with us. He was back at work in the driver's seat, and at his stop in front of the jail, he honked with one hand and stuck the other out the window to wave enthusiastically when he saw we had been released.

When those of us who had been arrested had our day in court, it was under the watchful eye of the late Justice Oscar Mitchell, whose portrait hung in the courtroom. Dr. Martin Luther King Jr., who had been arrested many times and sent to local jails often, was put into a maximum-security prison only once. Mitchell was the man who put him there.

One evening during the height of the civil rights movement, Dr. King was driving with his wife, Coretta Scott King, and Lillian Smith, a white activist and author who was in the passenger seat next to him. The police stopped them and arrested Dr. King, purportedly for driving with an Alabama license beyond the time when he should have acquired one from Georgia. Judge Mitchell sent King in the back of a police cruiser to Reidsville State Prison in the middle of the night. Fearing for his life, Mrs. King called U.S. Attorney General Bobby Kennedy, who intervened to get Dr. King freed.

As Judge Mitchell looked haughtily down upon us, our charges for interrupting the commission meeting with prayers and songs were dismissed. I imagine there was a disgusted harrumph from the old man, wherever he is.

At the next meeting of the DeKalb County Commission, several commissioners offered speeches to make emphatically clear that their decision to take a vote on the Grady funds had "nothing whatsoever to do with the demonstration" the previous week. Of course not. They approved the $1.1 million payment that was their obligation to the hospital. We thanked them and celebrated with gusto.

We were ready to tackle the state of Georgia next. We arranged a meeting with Democratic Governor Roy Barnes. He told us repeatedly that he was convinced of the essential role of Grady – not only for Atlanta but for the entire Southeast. As a Level 1 Trauma Center, and a designated Burn Center and Poison Control Center, Grady receives patients from around the state and beyond.

Gov. Barnes fussed and fumed about Grady's administrators, who could not manage to submit the correct paperwork for the state to make the required reimbursements. "Can't you do something to get them to *just send us the paperwork*," he pleaded, "so we can send the money over?" It was finally accomplished, and in the end Gov. Barnes allocated an additional $51 million for Grady's operations. It was a heady victory.

Over the years, we of the Open Door Community have been a part of many coalition efforts, but never one so widely diverse and energetic. While the *Atlanta Journal Constitution* refused to cover anything about the work of the Grady Campaign after the first march, the local television stations (especially Channel 11, the NBC affiliate) covered every action, every press conference, and the step-by-step progress of the effort. The TV news coverage generated even wider support and participation.

Unlike so much of what we're involved in on a day-to-day basis, this campaign, like the occupation of the Imperial Hotel, actually worked. Those of us who spend our time advocating for the homeless poor, prisoners, and those under death sentences are not accustomed to success. I'm still startled when I realize what we accomplished through the Grady Campaign. We changed hospital policy and helped preserve medical care for "zero card" patients at Grady. We were part of raising more than $58 million for the cash-strapped hospital in just four months and helped to avert an impending financial collapse. We were able to advocate for improvements in the pharmacy, so that it began serving clients more efficiently.

Part of the success of the Grady Coalition was based on the fact that at the core of the leadership was a group of us who had known and worked with each other for many years. A strong level of trust and mutual appreciation already existed, which enabled and empowered us to work together quickly to respond to the crisis. We created a very diverse coalition of individuals and groups working together in common cause. This challenged the popular assumption that we are a nation divided and segregated by race and class and other factors, and that there is very little we can do about it.

The Grady Coalition created a public experience of participatory democracy. The values and demands of the expanding global marketplace assume political lethargy from the general public. We are encouraged in our cynicism and distrust of what "government" can do about any of the problems we face. The more we believe that "we the people" are powerless to do what needs to be done, the more we are willing to turn over public business to private enterprise. In the process, the institutions of democracy and the democratic process itself suffer.

The Grady Coalition lifted a public clamor on behalf of the common good. We voted with our feet and our bodies and our voices, and we showed that it *can* be done: People *can* work together across all the walls that divide us and reshape the public agenda.

The dramatic public actions of the coalition planted seeds of imagination. All of us who witnessed the unfolding drama were encouraged in our faith and capacity to believe that the way things *are* is not the way things *have to be*. And our action spurred others to find their courage, to speak out and expose negligence and corruption. We experienced, you might say, a revival.

9

The Worst of Times

In May of 2001, the entire Open Door Community traveled to Greensboro, North Carolina, for Hannah's graduation from Guilford College. Six years before, I had been praying to live long enough to see my daughter graduate from high school. Being present to watch her walk across the stage and receive her college diploma was a poignant, shining moment. We reveled in a day of celebrating with Hannah and some of her best friends and professors. And I was thrilled that she had decided to spend the summer with us before moving to Philadelphia to take a job with *The Other Side*, a wonderful magazine that shared our commitments to faith, justice, and community.

That's about the only good thing I can say about 2001. I think I can honestly say that it was the worst year of my life.

In February the Open Door welcomed a couple that we came to see as "the volunteers from hell" – though of course at the time we did not know their point of origin. I'm not quite sure how we missed that they were not arriving among us bringing goodwill. We wrestled for a few months over asking them to leave – something we had to do occasionally when we were simply not able to integrate volunteers or guests into the unity of our shared life and work. Though we always tried to go about this difficult task with as little judgment as possible, we often failed to do it with enough grace and forgiveness. So the community decided over and over to keep trying to make things work with this couple – which we know in retrospect was a major mistake.

When summer rolled around, we filled the house with college-student volunteers. We liked them, but conflict arose quickly. The community gradually devolved into two distinct factions: those of us who lived there long-term and were stewards of the common life, and those who had come in as short-term volunteers. The visitors became more and more critical of those of us in the core community and complained about everything from our leadership style to Atlanta's sweltering summer heat.

Then we made another drastic mistake. We brought in a class from a local seminary to live, work, and study in the community for a week. Our requests that they prepare by reading some material we provided and that they leave behind items like their cars and credit cards were not honored. One student arrived in her shiny Cadillac and parked it among our dilapidated fleet, worrying aloud about whether it would be scratched or damaged.

When the class of all women began to settle in, a couple of them were clearly frightened and expressed distress about sleeping in rooms without locks. Though it was not said straight out, the concern was clearly related to sharing a household with so many poor people, especially African-American men. These students were ill-prepared to understand – let alone embrace – the diversity of our community, and we were wrong to swallow their insults.

Less than 48 hours after their arrival, the whole toxic mix exploded. We learned that the problem couple had been staying up late every night "debriefing" the college and seminary students and encouraging dissension, undermining our shared life. We found the clarity then to ask them to leave immediately, which just fueled the tension between us and the students. It was all a great and costly failure on our part, and the repercussions went on for years. We paid a high price for tolerating a destructive presence for far too long.

Community life depends on mutual openness, trust, and goodwill. It is always frustrating and sad when these are violated. At times we had to struggle greatly to keep our focus on the homeless poor and prisoners and not become resentful of those who had come to live with us but kept under the table their "exit strategy," made possible with abundant resources. The worst damage to the community has always been wreaked by people of privilege who come "half-way in" and leave when they find that those of us in the community are not only not saints, but are human beings with needs, wounds, and every imaginable variety of weakness and failing.

It was not clear how things could get worse. But they did. By late July I began having severe abdominal pain. I was in and out of the Grady Clinic, with no clarity about what the problem was. One afternoon I was sent to the emergency room thinking that the intestinal blockages had returned. But each time I moved into what seemed to be a crisis, the pain suddenly resolved itself. While trying to get an answer to this medical mystery, I lost a great deal of weight and felt awful most of the time.

At long last, in late September the doctors ordered a CAT scan. The "t" word was of course just what I didn't want to hear, but there it was: tumor. It was in my ileocecal valve, situated at the junction of my small and large intestines. This was the cause of the very painful swings in my gastrointestinal tract that had rendered me a physical wreck. I couldn't help noting the correspondence of my physical symptoms with the emotional turmoil of the community.

I needed surgery to remove the tumor, but first I needed a colonoscopy to determine its nature, to find out if it was malignant or benign. Again I ran up against a seemingly impenetrable wall at Grady. The Lower GI Clinic was backed up for more than six months, and I was informed that it would be several months before I could even call to make an appointment. This, of course, would only be tolerated in a poor peoples' hospital. Who with insurance and plenty of disposable income would tolerate being told that they could not even get on a waiting list for a procedure that the doctors had prescribed as desperately needed?

Ed and I began to pray for "a way out of no way." During our Open Door Sunday night worship service on October 14th, we prayed aloud for a pathway through this vexing problem. At supper after worship, we sat down with Jo, a young Open Door volunteer, and her mother, Susan Nicol. Jo moved away soon after that, and as far as I know that night was the first and only time Susan ever visited us at the Open Door.

As we ate, she said, "Tell me more about your need for a colonoscopy." I described my situation. She told us that she was the administrative assistant in the office of Emory Gastroenterology and worked with Dr. Vincent Yang, who performed the colonoscopies at Grady. Even though, she explained, people in need of one couldn't even get on a waiting list for six months, she offered to speak with him about my situation the next morning.

We of course could hardly believe what we were hearing. I'm aware that many people do not believe in prayer and surely not that

God answers prayers in a direct way. But if I ever had a doubt about the power of prayer before that night, it had vanished forever.

When I saw the primary care doctor in the Grady Clinic the next day, she came in with an astonished gasp: "Who do you know? *WHO do you know*?!" Her tone was a bit alarming. She couldn't believe that Dr. Yang was working me into his schedule the next day. "I can't get *any* of my patients into the Lower GI clinic!" she fumed. "How in the world did this happen?"

It was done. I had the colonoscopy. The faces around me were grim. "I don't know exactly what it is, but it's clearly malignant," reported the gastroenterologist. "Good thing you came when you did. You might have died if you had waited." This truth was truly stunning to me. If I had been a cooperative, "nice" patient and waited my turn, I most likely wouldn't have survived. I wondered how many Grady patients had died – and how many will yet die – waiting for a crucial diagnostic test. The tumor went off to the lab, and we waited.

On October 21st Ed and I drove to death row to be with our friend Terry Mincey, who was on "death watch." Being on death watch meant that a prisoner could have family and friends with him for the day before and the day of his execution, up until 3:00 p.m. I had been through death watch with friends on the row many times, spending hours caring for prisoners and their families and serving as a conduit to lawyers, at a moment of extreme anguish for everyone. Sometimes those hours seemed endless, and sometimes they seemed to fly by too quickly, as the clock ticked away the minutes until the state-imposed killing.

I had once emerged from a death watch with chest pains, and our wonderful pastoral counselor Dave Moylan told me, "You're not having a heart attack. Your heart is broken." Indeed, every death watch felt like an invitation to a broken heart.

That night Ed and I stayed at nearby New Hope House. In 1989, Mary Ruth and Ed Weir left Jubilee Partners in Comer, Georgia, with their young daughter Sabrina to found New Hope House. They were later joined by Lora and Bill Shain. Since 2015, the house has been directed by our wonderful friend Mary Catherine Johnson. New Hope House offers gracious hospitality to family and friends of death row prisoners when they make visits at the prison and, all too often, for the excruciating wait of death watch. As we had done many times before within its walls, we formed a small community of "hope beyond hope," praying for the unlikely possibility of a last-minute miracle. But at 7:00 p.m. on October 22nd, 2001, the state of Georgia took Terry's life.

Our friend Tamara Puffer had visited Terry for several years. We sat that night in the sadness with her and her partner Michael Galovic, who had lived with us for two years in the mid-1990s as an Open Door resident volunteer, and a few others who had gathered at New Hope House after the execution. The gloomy quiet was broken by the ringing telephone. My primary care doctor was calling. She had received the lab results from my colonoscopy: Burkitt's lymphoma.

I could hardly believe it. And apparently I wasn't alone. When my doctor spoke with my hematologist Jim Eckman, his response was, "Unheard of! This is 'write-uppable.' A recurrence of Burkitt's after six years? It just doesn't happen!" He said he would schedule surgery "right away."

The year 2001 had definitely started poorly, and it did not seem to be getting better.

"Right away" is different for Grady patients. The wait was hard, and I didn't make it to the scheduled surgery. On Saturday night, October 27th, the pain became unbearable as I grew weaker and more unable to tolerate food. Ed and Hannah, who was home for the weekend, drove me on the well-worn road to the Grady Emergency Room.

The first treatment was insertion of the dreaded NG tube to suction my stomach. "I need a 14French," I said as firmly as I could. The young resident looked at me coldly. I imagined what he was thinking: *And what do you know about the size of NG tubes? You're just a patient – and a Grady patient at that.*

To make things clear for him, I said, "I know that anything larger than a 14French is too large and causes constant pain." Having experienced the nightmare of an NG tube in 1995 that was the wrong size, I was very sure that I would stand my ground. He sighed and left the room.

When he came back he declared, "Well, we don't even have a 14French in the hospital."

"Then you're not putting an NG tube into me until you find one."

A little while later he returned with a 14French. The insertion was one of the worst medical procedures of my life – and that's saying something. He forced the tube up my nose and down my throat while I vomited over and over. When it was in, my throat felt like raw meat on the chopping block.

After this miserable procedure I was admitted to the fifth floor to await surgery. Soon, I had a few surprise visitors. Mr. Edward Renford, CEO of the hospital, came on my first day with an entourage of front-office folks. He said over and over, "If there's anything you need, Reverend Davis, you be sure to let us know." I'm certain he was imagining another protest line appearing in front of his hospital if anything went wrong with my care. One of the nurses was overheard asking, "Who *is* that in Room 505?" Apparently they had never before seen the CEO on their unit.

Tom Arrendale, a fellow Presbyterian and one of the vice presidents of the Grady Medical System, visited me nearly every weekday that I was there. Dr Curtis Lewis, our friend from the Interventional Radiology Department and Grady's medical director, came to check on me as well. We have never known anyone who loves Grady like Dr. Lewis. He was a very concerned, comforting presence. He assured us that he would be monitoring my care and the schedule for my surgery.

On Thursday we got word that I would have to wait until Monday for the surgery. It was one of the lowest points of my life. The raw pain in my throat was unabated – rivaling my abdominal pain. The agony was overwhelming me, and I was using every drop of physical and emotional energy just to endure from one hour to the next. I had no idea how I could hold on until Monday.

Dr. Lewis came by again that afternoon, and his brow furrowed when he heard about the schedule. A few hours later a nurse came in to tell me that I would be taken to surgery first thing the next morning. This was the second time on this journey that I received "special treatment." Thanks to my connections and the Grady Campaign, I was no ordinary Grady patient. Most patients do not have a direct link to get a colonoscopy when the waiting list is closed. Most do not receive personal visits from the CEO, vice president, and medical director of the hospital. And most needing to get into surgery right away do not have anyone to change the schedule on their behalf.

How to deal with this level of privilege? On the one hand, it was clear: I was suffering terribly. I was dying. I really *needed* these interventions. On the other hand, I had committed my life to solidarity with the poor. Should I just have kept my head under the radar and my mouth shut and accepted what would have been dealt to any other Grady patient?

I am not sorry for the preferential treatment. I believe I would have died without the intervention that got me in for a colonoscopy. I'm not sure what would have happened if I had been required to wait another three days for surgery. These interventions happened because of personal relationships. But the truth is that this is what *everybody* needs and deserves. I did not want preferential treatment, I wanted the treatment that each patient needs. What happened with me should not have been an aberration.

I have studied, meditated, and agitated since that moment about how we can move toward a standard of excellence in care for everyone, including the poorest and most vulnerable. Perhaps the most damning aspect of modern medicine is its de-personalization. Medical care is often seen as just one more transfer of capital, with patients referred to as "consumers." Taking human suffering and the need for healing – and paving it over with bureaucratic language that "manages" care as if healing is just one more function of the market – is obscene.

Personalism is a central value of the Catholic Worker life that the Open Door embraces. When someone is very sick, they need human beings with listening ears and hearts to say, "How can we help?" A depersonalized bureaucracy says, "No. No room for you. No, you cannot even get on a waiting list" – without even asking about the particulars of anyone's need. This is a system without a human heart, and it fuels the power of death and oppression.

Every Grady patient should have what I had: the concern and determination to make a way out of no way – not because I was a "VIP patient," as one administrator referred to me – but because every single patient is a human being who should be treated with utmost dignity, respect, and care. The word *hospital* is from the same root as *hospitality*, which might lead us to believe that in a hospital strangers and guests should be received with warmth, generosity, compassion – and, dare we say, with love?

So I am grateful for all that I received. But I hope never to take it for granted or to believe that I was in any way entitled to this special treatment. I was enormously thankful that I was pulled back from the brink of death yet again by the well-trained hands and hearts of healers. And I made an even deeper commitment to struggle for such care for all of our sisters and brothers at Grady, and wherever people reach out for healing.

That night the nurse was trying to insert a pre-surgery IV line. This was always difficult, because of the effect of chemo on my veins. She called in an IV specialist, but she also was unsuccessful. The specialist called in the resident, young Dr. Oberdeen, who was on the floor that night. He also failed. He told me grimly, "The only option left is to do a cut-down."

I shuddered. A cut-down is when a doctor cuts directly into the carotid artery in the neck to put in a central line. "I just don't want to do it," he said mercifully. "Even with a local anesthesia, it is very painful and difficult." He told me that he would leave it for the surgical team to put in an IV in the morning, or to do the cut-down after I was under general anesthesia. Fortunately, the next day someone from the team managed to get a line in a vein.

When I awoke from surgery, the sheet over my legs was rising and falling with the inflatable compression sleeves slipped over my legs, applying pressure through an air pump to improve my circulation and keep blood clots from forming. I lay there mesmerized by the movement when it dawned on me: *My NG tube is gone*! This was not typical after abdominal surgery. I gathered my wits and asked Ed why. He was delighted to see me coming back to consciousness and chuckled that this was my first question. "Yes," he said, "they took it out. They said that your throat was lacerated from the way they inserted it in the ER."

How hard I had to work not to say "I told you so!" I knew that night in the Emergency Room that the pain was simply worse than it should have been as the tube rubbed constantly against the shredded skin of my throat. The surgeons determined that it would be better for me to go without it than to make me continue to endure it. I was as grateful for this seemingly small consideration as for the removal of the awful tumor.

The surgeons had accessed my abdomen by cutting through the 23-inch scar left by my 1995 surgery. When my sister Dot heard that, she said, "Well gosh, why didn't they just put in a zipper?" We laughed and laughed.

But Ed and Hannah didn't think it was one bit funny. Usually they were the ones making me laugh, but this had been a rough go for them. They were more aware than I was at that point that the surgery behind me was just a small part of the medical drama that was to come. And it was exacerbated by more bad news from death row.

During the first week of my recovery, Jose High received a death warrant with an execution date. Jose was a generous soul – he had even somehow managed from death row to get flowers sent to my hospital room, with a sweet note in his own handwriting. We had known him for many years, and Ed was especially close to him. Their ways of looking at the world seemed to resonate in a unique way. We have a favorite Jose story – which is in fact a favorite among our many death row stories.

Jose suffered from obvious mental illness. As the date of his execution approached, the defense team hired a psychiatrist to come to the prison to do a professional evaluation. He performed many tests and talked with Jose at length. He wrote a comprehensive report for Jose's lawyers' use in the final appeals and clemency petition. Rachel Chmiel, one of the lawyers, had the task of going to the prison to meet with Jose and explain the report to him. At one point in the conversation Jose looked at Rachel and asked, "What exactly *is* mental illness?"

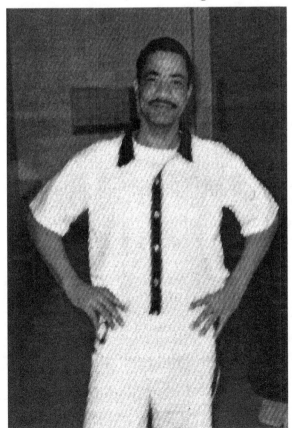

Jose High in his prison uniform in 2001. Photo by Wesley Baker, prison staff

Her mind quickly went into overdrive to come up with a way to put it, and then she gently explained. "Well, Jose, I guess you could say that it means your mind doesn't work quite like other people's minds."

Jose sat quietly, thinking about that for a moment. He smiled and nodded. And then he said, "Like Ed Loring. His mind doesn't work like other people's."

Rachel drove straight from the prison to the Open Door and found us at the dinner table. She couldn't wait to tell us about this exchange. We laughed about it loud and long. We're still laughing.

I was clearly unable to go anywhere – much less to death row – and Ed was reluctant to leave me. But we all knew that Jose needed him at the prison. So while I worked to make it through each hour, Ed – along with Rachel, Mary Sinclair, and Ellie Hopkins from Jose's legal team – traveled back and forth between my hospital room and the visiting room at death row. They left him just before his execution, plunged into deep grief as they walked out of the prison with Jose's loving daughter.

Two days after Jose's death, Ed got a call from Chaplain John Mohammed, asking if he could come and talk with us. Jose had asked this greatly trusted Muslim chaplain at the prison to be with him at the time of his execution. Chaplain Mohammed arrived in my hospital room still shaken by his experience and in deep need of talking with long-time friends who could understand his anguish. He told us that what he had witnessed was barbaric. "I was in Vietnam," he said, "and I *never* saw anything worse than this."

The prison's IV execution team had had difficulty finding a good vein in which to insert the needle to conduct the lethal drugs that would kill Jose. His veins too were broken down by early years of IV drug use. The team tried over and over, sticking needles into various parts of his body with no success. As the time of the scheduled execution approached, they decided to perform a cut-down. I shuddered again as Chaplain Mohammed said, "They proceeded without anesthesia."

Apparently unfazed by Jose's groans and screams, the so-called medical team cut open his neck, got the line placed in his carotid artery, and then killed Jose right on schedule. Of course nothing was publicly reported about what they did or how they did it. No one ever mentioned Jose's extreme suffering. No one accused the Department of Corrections of willful torture or violating the Constitution's Eighth Amendment prohibiting cruel and unusual punishment.

No responsible doctor or medical technician would ever think of performing a cut-down in a non-emergency situation, and certainly not without appropriate anesthesia. I was spared that agony by a caring young doctor because I was among healers; Jose had to endure it because he was in the hands of butchers. We know that a person cannot agree to be a professional killer without having already sunk into barbarism; and once death is the goal, anything can happen along the way. We learned a lot that day about the lengths to which de-sensitized prison employees will go to "get the job done" – even when "the job" is killing one of the people in their care.

The following week, I had to have another PAS port surgically implanted in my right upper arm for the administration of my chemotherapy. I was taken again to Interventional Radiology, where the technicians strapped my right arm onto an extender attached to the surgical table. Dr. Peters, the radiologist, swabbed my arm in preparation for the anesthesia, but then she was called away for an emergency. With my arm strapped down, unable to move my body for about an hour and a half, I waited.

That time on the table was one of the extraordinarily rare moments when I was absolutely alone, and it prompted some of the most intense reflection I have ever experienced. I was in a darkened, quiet room. Tears began to pool in my eyes as I realized that, only a few days earlier, Jose had been strapped to an almost identical table, with both of his arms lashed to extenders, his body arrayed in the form of a cross. I never felt so close to my friends on death row. I felt like I was "one" with them.

But our physical position had opposite meaning for us. I was strapped down waiting for someone to cut my arm and insert needles. So were my friends. But they waited for needles that would cause suffering, harm, and death. I waited for needles that were intended for healing, good, and restoration of life. They were subjected to crucifixion, and I was on the way to resurrection.

"Hoelzer" was the chemotherapy regimen the doctors agreed on. Drs. Jim Eckman and Sid Stein were my attending hematologists, and I had three hematology fellows: Jawan Ayer-Cole, Martha Arellano, and Michael Benjamin. Jawan and Martha were regularly in and out of my room, and I looked forward to their visits. Martha remains a friend whom Ed and I saw often after she became an associate professor of hematology and oncology at Emory's Winship Cancer Center.

The regimen was, they explained to me, one of the most complex and rigorous treatments available. I was to be hospitalized for each treatment for a week to 10 days, and during that time I would be in isolation. I could expect to be sick in the wake of each treatment, but they were hopeful that the aggressive regimen would put the lymphoma back into remission.

Nothing, however, could have prepared me for the months that were to come. I spent a total of 89 days and nights on the 10th-floor oncology ward – most of that time in one of the three isolation units. After most of the seven- to 10-day cycles I got very sick, and many times Ed had to get up with me in the middle of the night to rush me to the Emergency Room with a high fever. There I would be admitted again to the hospital, where the doctors launched an assortment of broad-spectrum antibiotics coursing through my bloodstream.

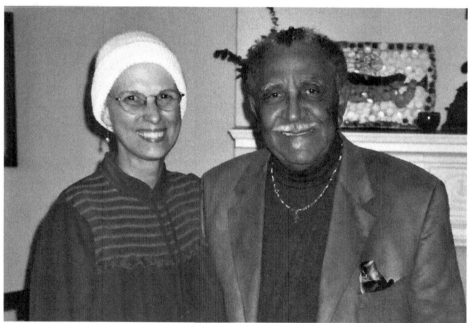

Rev. Dr. Joseph Lowery, a dear friend and civil rights icon, came by for a pastoral visit in 2002. Photo by Hannah Loring-Davis

Never did I have to be so vigilant about my chemotherapy. Increased budget cuts at Grady meant drastic cuts in staff as well, and nurses who should have been overseeing treatment for one patient were caring for many. No one can do this responsibly, and I knew competent and caring nurses on the oncology floor who quit or requested a move to another part of the hospital, out of fear of being responsible for the death of a chemo patient.

As a patient receiving the Hoelzer regimen, I knew that I would have to be "in charge" of my own care. I often refrained from taking medication to relieve the pain, because I had to be alert to ensure that my drugs were administered correctly. As Ed and I had in 1995, after getting Methotrexate I set an alarm clock at six-hour intervals so that I would receive the rescue drug Leucovorin on time and avoid kidney, liver, or heart damage. In the hospital, it came infused through my IV tube rather than in pill form. At times I had to call the nurses' station in the middle of the night to insist that it was time for the drug. Sometimes I had to argue until it arrived. I suspect I was considered a demanding patient, but I understood that my life was at stake.

I again thought often of the many Grady patients I had met who didn't possess the education or nerve to direct their own care. When I completed this complex chemotherapy regimen in the spring of 2002, I spoke with Drs. Eckman and Stein, strongly encouraging them to transfer any Grady patient needing the Hoelzer regimen to Emory. I was relieved and grateful that they agreed and changed hospital policy.

I walked the narrow border between life and death at many points. I would not have endured without Ed and Hannah. I am forever grateful that our generous friends Dee Dee Rischer and Will O'Brien of *The Other Side* magazine freed up Hannah to make frequent trips from Philadelphia to Atlanta. The love that closed in to help us through this second journey seemed to me as healing as the medical interventions. The treatment this time made 1995 seem like a picnic; some days I wasn't sure if the doctors were trying to get me well or just kill me outright. But I never doubted the loving care that buoyed Ed, Hannah, and me as we stumbled along this treacherous path.

Friends Elizabeth Dede, Denise Ghee, and Mary Ruth Weir spent long, sleepless nights with me, giving Ed a break and a chance to get some rest. Nan and Erskine Clark visited, cooked, and tended to us. Mary Sinclair, Joyce Hollyday, and sister Dot visited regularly. Every Sunday night a community member, often Dick Rustay, brought us communion after worship. Lee Miller and Bob Eckhardt, both deacons at St. Anne's Episcopal Church, brought us the Eucharist on several occasions as well, along with delicious meals. We had a wonderful visit with Jeff Dietrich and Catherine Morris, long-time members of the Los Angeles Catholic Worker, who came all the way from the west coast.

We were touched by visits from even farther away. Our dear friend, German theologian Jürgen Moltmann, always came to see us at the Open Door when he was in Atlanta delivering lectures at Emory's Candler School of Theology, which happened rather frequently. Sometimes his partner, Elisabeth, accompanied him, and Ed and I visited them once in their home in Tübingen, Germany. Whenever I was in the hospital, he visited me there. On his visit the following spring, he gave me his cherished pocket Bible with this inscription: *My pocket Bible, to Murphy, with all my hope, in constant prayer. Jürgen, April 8, 2002.* It remains a treasured gift.

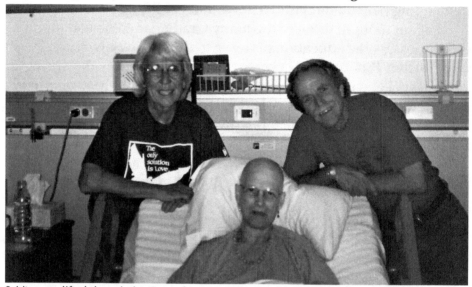

Spirits were lifted through the times of treatment by the visits of friends from far and near. Catherine Morris and Jeff Dietrich came from the Los Angeles Catholic Worker in the spring of 2002 and brought laughter, prayers, and deep friendship, representing the ongoing presence of the wide Catholic Worker network in the life of the Open Door Community. Photo by Ed Loring

I got another special gift that year. I had worked closely for many years with Charlotta Norby and her partner, Steve Bright, both renowned anti-death-penalty lawyers. After Charlotta experienced a brain aneurism, she had to give up her legal work and took up quilting. She gave me one of her beautiful, specially created quilts, made up of squares depicting things and events that were dear to me, like a guitar and a picket line.

One morning a nurse took a look at it spread out on my hospital bed, smiled, and said, "Oh, it's so pretty. It's so nice of your friend to make this for you." Then she stopped, got a disbelieving look on her face, and said, "Ms. Davis, there's a toilet on your quilt."

I hastily explained that since homeless people were regularly imprisoned in the Atlanta City Jail for the "crime" of public urination, we had maintained a steady campaign for public toilets in Atlanta over a period of many years.

Billy Neal Moore also visited. I first met him on death row in 1978, and we quickly became very close. In 1979, when I was pregnant with Hannah, Billy wrote to me that before he went to sleep each night, he held his pillow very carefully, pretending it was the baby. He was very concerned that he might not remember how to hold an infant and wanted to greet the baby with all the tenderness he had to give. I brought Hannah to meet him when she was six weeks old. Billy held and cuddled her like the experienced parent he was to his son, Little Billy.

Twice I went through death watch with Billy. Each time he was put into the cell next to the electric chair and left there with two guards, to count down the hours until his execution. I was with him first in 1984 for the excruciating tick-tock of the prison's *danse macabre*. As we sat in the small visiting room, the prison riot squad came and went, clattering their military boots and paraphernalia through the cell blocks to threaten and intimidate. The front office men assembled and dispersed, looking officious and grim as ashes. Most guards looked away, but a few looked at Billy sympathetically, and some even spoke words of greeting. They all knew that Billy was a good man who made their jobs easier by keeping peace on the row.

Billy made it through both times. Eventually, with the pleas of many, including the victim's family, he not only left death row after 16 years, he was paroled to the "free world" in 1991. And then (miraculously), he was even freed from parole. He was ordained as a minister and has travelled far and wide to tell his story in law schools and churches, to students and advocacy groups.

As I had sat with him fighting for his life as the hours crept toward death, there was Billy with his wife and clergy partner, Donna, sitting in my hospital room, talking and praying, fighting for mine. It was a glorious circle of life and hope. Who could have dreamed it?

As Christmas came close, I fretted about how to get 115 packages ready for our friends on death row. Charlotta , Mary Sinclair, and Anne Wheeler, who generously helped to guide the administrative work of the Open Door, stepped up and got it done. But Gladys Rustay knew that I was suffering to be stuck in bed while my friends did the work that had been such a joy to me for so many years. So she planned a party.

Gladys and Dick Rustay could always be counted on to do whatever needed to be done at the Open Door. When co-founders Carolyn and Rob Johnson left the community after a few years, we ran a free "want ad" in *Sojourners* magazine. We explained that we needed volunteers and blankets for our work with homeless people. The best response we got was from Dick.

Having regional leadership responsibilities with the childhood development agency Head Start, Dick traveled from Asheville, North Carolina, and spent two days in Atlanta every week. Instead of staying in a nice hotel, he decided that he could spend a night at our shelter, making dinner and cookies in the evening and breakfast in the morning, shaving in the shared public bathroom before going off to his meetings. Over the years he and Gladys, a kindergarten teacher, visited us often at the Open Door, especially around holidays, and their son Chris and daughter Kim spent time with us as resident volunteers. In 1989 they retired, sold their home in Asheville, and joined the community in September.

Gladys set up a table right outside our apartment door, with hot cider, cookies, and other goodies. Christmas music played on the boom box, and several friends came over. It was beautiful, but I was already crashing toward bottom. By the time Gloria Lee and Sarah Fitten, beloved friends from the Grady Campaign, came by with gifts and sweet hugs, I could feel my fever rising above the danger point of 101.5 degrees. From long experience, I had become an expert at knowing exactly when I had to show up in the Emergency Room. I wanted so badly to be part of the Christmas cheer, but I pulled on Ed's shirt sleeve and whispered with dismay, "We've got to go to the hospital."

That's when I realized that 2001 was going to end as badly as it had started.

It always took hours to get seen in the Emergency Room, but the staff never failed to get me quickly into a room isolated from the throng of coughing, bleeding, groaning patients. Chemotherapy killed off many of my infection-fighting white blood cells called neutrophils, and after every treatment I was vulnerable to every sort of bacteria. I was at risk of entering the danger zone of neutropenia, with too few neutrophils to fight off infections – a serious, even deadly, threat.

Indeed, I had once again developed a serious but unidentified infection, so the doctors ordered another round of powerful doses of IV antibiotics. I was way down in the dumps – sick as I could be, with everybody around me worried – and it was Christmas, for heaven's sake! Though I loathe all the consumeristic hype of Christmas, I love the liturgy of Advent, I love the music, and I love the way we celebrate the season with our friends who are homeless and in prison. It leaves very little time or energy for attention to exchanging gifts among people who don't need anything.

It turned out that I was also anemic, so the doctors ordered several units of packed red blood cells for a transfusion. The transfusion started while my sister Dot was visiting the next day. She said later, "It was like watching you come back to life. As the blood flowed into your arm, I watched the color come back into your face and the energy back to your tired, slumping body." During transfusions I always felt like a wilted flower being thrust at last into fresh water, feeling my drooping leaves and petals begin to rise and bloom again. I was revived and sent home.

I have received gallons and gallons of packed red blood cells and platelets over the years. And I've thought often of Blanche Dubois in Tennessee Williams' *A Streetcar Named Desire*, declaring in her distinctive, syrupy, Southern drawl: "I have always depended on the kindness of strangers." Thanks to the kindness of strangers, I must by now have the blood of every race and class and age of people flowing through my veins. I am more grateful than I can say for everybody who extends an arm to give blood. Time and again my life has depended on this kindness – creating in me not only gratitude, but an embodied solidarity, circulating in my deepest self. A Christmas gift beyond measure.

The transfusion gave me the energy to enjoy a visit from my Dad, who traveled from High Point, North Carolina, just before Christmas. He stayed with Dot in nearby Decatur, and we were all grateful for a warm and wonderful Christmastime together. But the good tidings didn't last long. Just when we thought nothing else could go wrong, I had to be readmitted to Grady the day after Christmas – and on that same day my Dad had a heart attack. Suddenly Dot was getting an ambulance to rush him to DeKalb Medical Center, the closest hospital to her home. She spent the rest of that week shuttling back and forth between the two hospitals – one day even taking Polaroid photos of each of us to take to the other.

CHAPTER 9

When Dad was stabilized, Dot had to arrange medical transport to get him back to his room in the Presbyterian Home in High Point. He lived another year and a half, but his traveling days were done. Though his physical strength never returned after the heart attack, his spirit in his last months was as sweet and loving as we had always known it to be. He died at 10:30 in the morning on Easter Sunday in 2003 – just in time to make it to church in heaven, we always joked.

Ed and I spent the end of 2001 confined to an isolation unit at Grady. It was definitely not where we wanted to ring in the New Year, but it seemed fitting that such an awful year would end there. I'm sure we were feeling sorry for ourselves, lamenting all that 2001 had put us through. New Year's Eve on the cancer ward was, shall we say, a bit on the morose side.

But as the evening wore on, the door swung open and a young Russian resident who was receiving her training at Grady floated in. I wish I could remember her name, but it was a long Russian one, and everyone always referred to her simply as Dr. Sky.

To celebrate New Year's Eve on the cancer ward, Dr. Sky had baked a special Russian honey cake for her co-workers, made of more layers than I had the energy to count, with sweet cream frosting between each. She handed a huge piece to Ed and me – a slice of exquisite, delicious kindness. It was utter perfection – a finishing note of grace that enabled us to say that, for one brief moment, our horribly dreadful year ended well.

10

Crossing Over and Back

By the spring of 2002, I began to anticipate the joy of finishing the horrific Hoetzler regimen. Our good friend Norman Shanks, leader of the Iona Community in Scotland, invited Ed and me to come in late June to teach a course with him. We were very excited about the possibility of a trip to the beautiful Isle of Iona, a small island in the Inner Hebrides off Scotland's west coast, and to share time with that wonderful community and its associates who would converge from around the world for a summer gathering. But we knew we couldn't say a definite yes until we saw how my post-chemo recovery would go.

It was no small shock when I was in the clinic in April and Drs. Eckman and Ayer-Cole sat down to talk with us. "You're doing so well that we want to transfer you to Emory to have a bone marrow transplant as soon as you've finished the last dose of chemotherapy," Dr. Eckman said. It took a lot of time and explanation for us to catch up with their thinking.

Only Dr. Stein, we later learned, had serious reservations about my undergoing the transplant. "She's had to suffer so much," he explained to Ed. "I just don't want to see her have to go through this." Tears were seeping out of the corners of his eyes as he said it.

But after extensive conversations, it was decided that we should pursue the transplant. The planning began, and as soon as I finished chemo Ed and I went to Emory's Winship Cancer Center to meet Dr. Istvan Redei, a hematologist. He spoke with a thick Hungarian accent and moved briskly, and he presented us with truckloads of information about what would be coming.

The first task was to ask my sister and brothers to be tested, to see if one of them would be a match. A sibling match is considered the best for an allogeneic transplant, which involves taking the bone marrow or stem cells from a donor and grafting them to the cancer patient's blood system. The docs were delighted that I had three possible donors. Dot and my brothers Mac and Les didn't hesitate to step up, but unfortunately none was a match. When the results were in, I remarked to them, "We've always said that the four of us are really different from each other – and *now* we've got genetic proof."

The medical staff was deeply disappointed. The next step was to pursue an autologous transplant, involving harvesting peripheral stem cells from my own blood, purging them with the drug Rituxan, and then freezing them. After more rounds of chemotherapy to essentially obliterate my immune system, the stem cells would be infused back into my blood, to graft and re-create a healthy, cancer-free system.

Throughout my recent chemo treatment, I had given myself daily shots of Neupogen (also known as Filgrastim) in my abdomen. Neupogen is a laboratory-created form of a protein that stimulates the growth of white blood cells in the body after they have been destroyed by chemotherapy. To continue building up my white cells and mobilizing stem cells, I ramped up the Neupogen injections to twice a day. Every few days I was tested to see how my stem cells were coming along.

After two rigorous weeks of tests, pokes, prods, blood draws, injections, infusions, and educational sessions, Dr. Redei called us into his office. He cut to the chase. "Your body has had so much chemotherapy that you do not have enough stem cells for a transplant," he said. "You have enough to keep a reasonably healthy blood supply, but none to spare." He explained that the only remaining transplant option was an allogeneic transplant from an anonymous donor. "But this is far too risky, and we would not do this unless your life is at stake," he said. "So, that's it. You should just be as careful as you can, and try to stay healthy. If the lymphoma comes back, we will pursue an anonymous donor transplant. Good luck." He shook our hands and was gone.

My elbow was in Ed's ribs. "Hey," I said with more energy than I had felt in many moons, "let's go to Scotland!"

"*What?*" He looked at me entirely baffled. I had sort of figured that Dr. Redei's news was coming, but Ed had been caught completely off guard, and he was in no way prepared for my reaction to it.

"Scotland!!" I said. "Let's call Norman and tell him we can come!"

"Oooh!" It finally came together in Ed's mind. We went home and made the call. By that evening, we were booking our flights.

When we arrived at the Shanks' home on Iona in late June, I was skinny and bald, with pasty skin. I was so weak I could barely walk around the block. But our two weeks there were nothing if not idyllic. Norman and Ruth are great friends, and Ed and I were ready to have a good time. Uncharacteristically for Scotland, the sun shone almost every day.

We ate well, including of course tea time every afternoon – with tea, cookies, and *chocolate*! We walked everywhere on this small island that allowed only a few cars. We taught the course, and I even preached at the Iona Abbey Church one Sunday – one of the great honors of my life. After two weeks I had "roses in my cheeks," I had put on a little weight, and on one of our last days there I walked six miles. I had come back to life in the sunshine and glorious fresh salt air of that beautiful island.

My relatively good health lasted for two years. After a routine PET scan in the spring of 2004, Rick White, the nurse coordinator at my clinic, called to tell me I needed to come in. I knew from something in his voice that he was upset, and I figured bad news was on the way. But I couldn't be sure until Ed and I were in the clinic and heard it from my docs, and I didn't want to worry anyone needlessly, so I kept my concern to myself.

Dr. Jim Eckman, steady, brilliant, trustworthy, compassionate senior physician, sat down and broke the news about the spread of my lymphoma. "The nodes are all over your chest – around your lungs and a number in your abdomen." He looked directly at me with kindness. "So," he said, "you know what's next?" It was clear that the bone marrow transplant was back on the table, and almost before I could answer him, he sent his colleague Dr. Benjamin down the hall to call Dr. Sagar Lonial at Emory, to get things started.

It was starting all over again. Because I had some idea that something like this was coming, I wasn't devastated by the news. Ed, on the other hand, was totally unprepared and had tears streaming down his face. Dr. Eckman's eyes fixed on Ed. "Look after this guy," he said to me, his hand on Ed's shoulder.

We knew that the bone marrow transplant from an anonymous donor would be the greatest challenge I had faced yet. Survival was by no means assured. And if I did survive, I was almost certain to face graft-versus-host disease (GVHD). While the donor would be as close a match as possible, the transplanted immune cells in the tissue (the graft) would nevertheless recognize me (the host) as "foreign." The graft would then likely attack my body cells, causing illness or disorders of the liver, skin, mucosal membranes, gastrointestinal tract, connective tissue, and/or lungs. Some of the potential reactions of GVHD are truly horrifying.

We needed the help of a wise spiritual guide to face this new challenge. For years we had depended on Anthony Granberry, a pastoral counselor with special training in addiction, to offer guidance for our common life – especially as we served and shared life with so many people struggling with chemical dependency. At this critical juncture, the community needed a word from him. We invited him to preach the following Sunday.

Anthony minced no words. His sermon was titled "Faith or Fear." He unabashedly claimed my healing. He declared that we had a clear choice: to go into my next medical adventure with fear – or to claim our faith and walk with strength, in the confidence that what we needed would be provided. He confessed to me later that he was somewhat anxious about claiming healing before the horrendous treatment had even begun; but he felt "mysteriously compelled" and knew that he must be faithful to the word that had come to him. His words stayed alive in our hearts through the long, hard days…and weeks…and months that followed.

Dr. Lonial met Ed and me at the Emory Winship Cancer Clinic and reviewed with us the basics of the bone marrow transplant process. I checked into Emory Hospital on June 15 for Round 1, Part A, of another killer chemo regimen, called Hyper C-Vad, so that I would be ready in the event that a matching donor was found. The radiologist inserted a Hickman catheter into a large vein in my upper chest, to carry drugs directly into my heart and from there all over my body. A large, triangular, plastic contraption hung from my chest, and three plastic catheters hung almost to my waist – a most annoying arrangement.

Dr. Amelia (Amy) Langston, director of the Bone Marrow Transplant Center, walked into my room that day with my medical chart under her arm and introduced herself to Ed and me. She spoke in low tones – until she was clear that we were aware of the gravity of my situation. Then, she looked straight at me and said point-blank: "You *know* you're not supposed to be alive, don't you?"

Her question hung in the air for a split second and then all three of us burst into laughter. "Thanks for showing us your best bedside manner from the get-go!" I said. That exchange sealed the friendship that endures to the present. Gratefully, I remained under Amy's care for the next 13 years. Ed and I even had the honor of traveling to Washington state in 2013 to officiate at the wedding of Amy and her partner, Beverlee Silva. Bev's mother was dying, and they wanted to get married while she was still able to share the joy with them. It was a beautiful and poignant celebration.

Another beautiful thing came out of this new crisis. The challenge of finding a donor for an allogenic transplant was taken up by Hannah, Mary Sinclair, and Lauren Cogswell. Lauren, a Presbyterian minister who faithfully brought me the Eucharist during my hospitalization, had volunteered at the Open Door for several years and then spent five years living with us as a resident volunteer and leader. They got all the information they needed from Be the Match, which under the auspices of the National Marrow Donor Program has for the last 30 years managed the world's largest and most diverse bone marrow registry.

Testing is done today by swabbing the inside of a potential donor's cheek, but back then it required drawing blood. After my first round of chemo, Hannah, Mary, and Lauren hosted a big party at the Open Door. A nurse came and took blood from any and all volunteers, so that their information could be entered into the registry. The hope was always that new volunteers would match me or somebody else who needed a transplant. Scores of friends and co-workers came to hold out their arms and sign up: Open Door volunteers, lawyers and staff from the Southern Center for Human Rights and the Georgia Resource Center, friends from churches and law firms in the city, and people we had never before met or seen.

It spread out from there. Many local churches and Columbia Theological Seminary set up their own bone marrow registry drives. Former Open Door volunteers Joseph and Suzanne Hobby Shippen held a drive at General Theological Seminary in New York, where Joseph was studying for the Episcopal priesthood. And former resident volunteers Robbie Turner and Melissa Genord organized one in Lexington, Kentucky.

CHAPTER 10

We all knew that there were many cancer patients who needed transplants but found no match. The need was most critical for African Americans. My nurse practitioner, Janet Lee, told us about one of her patients who was ready for a transplant but waited and waited. Finally, a match came, but after much excitement, the donor backed out. A second match was found, and again, the donor declined. Her patient died. Janet was filled with grief, and my "team" worked especially hard to find African-American donors. As time went on, it became less about just my need for a donor and more about all of the people out there who needed, and were less likely to find, a match. This, of course, was a joy to me.

The best successes came many months after my transplant process was set aside. Mary lined up contacts at the Fulton County Government Center and Atlanta City Hall. The majority of workers in both buildings are African American, and the drives were very successful. It was a wonderful gift of solidarity for these dear friends and family to work so long and tirelessly – stirred by my need, but working in a way that gave hope for a match to many others who suffered with cancer.

Grace abounded in all corners. Our dear friend Al Winn, a courageous retired Presbyterian leader living in Winston-Salem, North Carolina, wrote to us, indignant that his doctor told him that he could not be my donor. No one over the age of 60 is allowed to donate, but Al tried hard to get the rules bent.

Marietta Jaeger-Lane, whose 7-year-old daughter Susie had been kidnapped during a family camping vacation and murdered, wrote from Montana. Marietta co-founded Journey of Hope for murder victims' families opposed to the death penalty, and she had stayed at the Open Door years before during a march through Georgia. She described it in her letter to me as "a blest time in a sacred space." She explained that her younger sister had been diagnosed with leukemia, and Marietta was the only sibling who was a match for a bone marrow transplant. She included copies of her medical and lab reports, offering, "If any of this is of value and subsequent use for you, Murphy, I'd be honored and privileged to share my bone marrow with you."

I received letters from many friends in prison who wanted to be tested. Most touching was a letter from an intellectually disabled man on death row who asked the guards and administration every day to let him give me his bone marrow. By the end of his letter to me, it became clear that he believed that donating his bone marrow to me would cost him his own life – but it was what he wanted to do more than anything.

In July I returned for Round 1, Part B, of my chemotherapy. On the day I was admitted, Dr. Christopher Flowers, a brilliant young African-American physician, came into my room and handed me a list of the chemo drugs, carefully going over each, stopping to ask if I had questions or concerns as he went along. Once again I kept the list of drugs and the order of their administration in my notebook on the table by my bed.

When a nurse came in to give me an IV, I asked her what was in the bag. When she said Rituxan, I said, "I'm so sorry, but this is not on the list of drugs I got from Dr. Flowers." She arched her eyebrows, turned, and left the bag hanging on my pole as she briskly left the room. Later Dr. Flowers came back through the door laughing. "You caught me, Ms. Davis, and you're right," he said. "I didn't tell you about the Rituxan, and you proved you were listening carefully." He explained that Rituxan is not technically a chemotherapy drug, so it wasn't on the list. "But it *is* an important part of your treatment," he emphasized. He laughed again. "I told the nurses, 'Remember, Ms. Davis is a Grady patient.'"

I was learning what it was like to be in a cancer center with a full, experienced staff. And I began to relax in a way I had never experienced before while getting chemotherapy. I kept my little notebook, but I began to trust the process more than I had ever dreamed possible. And I wished for the day when the level of care provided at Emory will be the standard we demand for everybody – including the poorest of the poor.

Over the years, through my encounters with Burkitt's lymphoma, I learned more about the disease that was pursuing me – and the Irish gastroenterologist who identified it in 1958. While he was serving in Africa, Dr. Denis Burkitt discovered that Ugandans – who ate an extraordinarily high-fiber, plant-based diet – had an almost non-existent rate of colon cancer. He universally recommended such a diet and was acclaimed as the first medical scientist to recognize the importance of dietary fiber in the prevention of colon cancer.

Also while in Uganda, Dr. Burkitt began seeing men and boys with tumors in their mouths, jaws, and necks. He knew that their condition was fatal without treatment and secured permission to administer the drug Cytoxan (Cyclophosphamide). Noticeable shrinkage took place in the tumors of his patients who received the infusions. Some went into remission, and some were even cured.

As with all experimental drugs, risk and courage were called for on the part of both doctor and patients on the way to determining doses and limits. Almost four decades later, I received Cytoxan during my first chemotherapy regimen – and I eventually reached my "lifetime limit" of the drug. I owe my life in part to the bravery of men and boys in Africa – some of whom surely gave their lives on the way to discovering the limit – and to the compassionate wisdom of Dr. Burkitt.

While I was deep into my perilous journey toward a bone marrow transplant in 2004, I received an email out of the blue from an Irish woman named Mary, who said that a friend of hers had told her about my long struggle with Burkitt's lymphoma and had explained that I was again very ill and in rigorous treatment. She wrote: *I wanted to write to tell you that Dr. Denis Burkitt was my very good friend. He was a wonderful humble Christian man who made great contributions to the faith and medical advances around the world...Denis' widow, Olive Burkitt, is alive and well. I have told her about you and your illness. She is praying for your health, along with your family, and I am praying for you as well.* How I wish I still had that e-mail so that I could tell her how much it has meant to me over the years.

Dr. George McCloud, Scottish pastor and founder of the Iona Community, said on at least one occasion, "If you believe in coincidence, you deserve a very boring life." I think McCloud was right, and that much of what is dismissed as "coincidence" is the providence of God. Sometimes it's palpable. I have come to understand and define providence as the loving, liberating power of God woven through all of life and creation and history – which, as the apostle Paul put it in his letter to the Roman church, brings "all things [to] work together for good for those who love God" (Rom. 8:28).

I never *wanted* to have cancer. I never desired to be critically ill or to walk the razor's edge between life and death. I would never say that it was a good thing that I have gone through the illness I have faced and survived. But, oh, the miracles of love and goodness that have emerged every step of the way!

How, otherwise, could I explain such an unlikely connection with the family of the physician who identified and began to treat the awful cancer that continued to attack my body? How to account for such love reaching across an ocean and a culture to extend a word of friendship and love and the assurance of prayers and support? How else could it be that a terrible disease became the vehicle of friendship, solidarity, and the "fleshing out" of the Mystical Body of Christ that reaches into every corner of the earth?

Another great gift appeared on our doorstep that summer. Our dear friends Nelia and Calvin Kimbrough, who were among the co-founders of the Patchwork Central community in Evansville, Indiana, and had lived there for 27 years, decided to move to Atlanta and join us at the Open Door. When Ed got Calvin's phone call with this

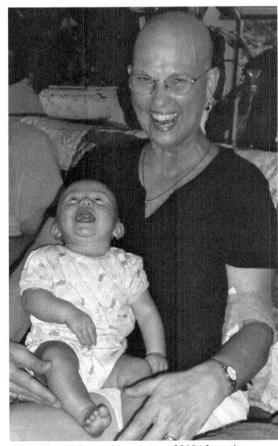

A special visit during the summer of 2004 from three-month-old John Thomas Loring, who had just learned to giggle and made his grandmother's heart glad. Photo by Diane Wiggins

news, he was so excited and flabbergasted that he hung up the phone to tell me – without offering a word of response to Calvin. It remains a source of laughter between the four of us to this day. When Calvin and Nelia heard how sick I was, they stepped up their arrival date by a few weeks and came to us in August.

Both ordained United Methodist pastors, Nelia is an extraordinary artist and liturgist, and Calvin an outstanding photographer and banjo player who is also the layout editor for *Hospitality*. I first met them in the early 1970s, when Nelia was named the first coordinator of women's programming at Emory's Candler School of Theology. It was an era when feminist theology was just beginning to be recognized. No women served on the faculty of any of Atlanta's seminaries, and few were students. So, in order to have a "critical mass," Nelia and I worked to get together women from Candler, Columbia Theological Seminary, and the Interdenominational Theological Center. Walt Lowe, a very supportive Candler professor, wryly commented on our effort, "And they were a *very* critical mass."

After completing another round of chemo in August, I immediately began to feel very weak. I even fainted at the wedding of Amy Vosburg and Mike Casey. Fortunately, I waited until just after they had exchanged their vows. Amy was a lawyer with the Georgia Appellate Research Center, working on cases of death row prisoners, and Mike, who had lived with us as a resident volunteer from 2001 to 2003, worked with the Georgia Justice Project, where they had met. Their wedding was a joyous occasion, and I hated becoming the center of attention on a day that should have been theirs alone.

I was sitting in a wheelchair when I lost consciousness. Hannah and our beloved friend Heather Bargeron, who had lived with us off and on for a decade and faithfully worked on *Hospitality*, were singing in the choir and rushed immediately to my side. Ed stood and asked, "Is there a doctor in the house?" Dan Casey, a physician – who also happened to be Mike's brother and the best man in the wedding – carefully tended to me. When I was wheeled out, I waved, embarrassed, and everyone clapped. Ed kissed Amy on the cheek on the way out the door – announcing with a grin "I was the first to kiss the bride!" – and then whisked me straight to Emory Hospital.

I was sure I was in the neutropenic zone again, and tests confirmed it. In the days that followed, we were, as always, very careful. "Hand hygiene saves lives," Hannah pronounced in a singsong voice as she came and went, echoing the words of the sign that was posted everywhere in the Bone Marrow Transplant Unit at the hospital and in the Emory Clinic. We took it very seriously. We believed it, practiced it, and we continue to be ridiculously scrupulous about it.

I always tried not to do stupid things when I was neutropenic, and Ed was a hawk. Nobody came near me without thoroughly washed hands. No kisses, and very few hugs. No raw fruits or vegetables – only well-cooked foods to kill any surface bacteria. And gifts of fresh flowers or potted plants had to be turned away at our apartment door and enjoyed by the rest of the community downstairs.

But bacteria, viruses, and fungi are omnipresent. Amy Langston told us, "Well, you can only be so careful. This stuff is in the air. You breathe it – inside and out. When you have a healthy immune system, you fight it off. When you're neutropenic, it comes after you."

And so it happened that a fungus floated through the air and settled into my lungs. When? Where? How? Why? Useless to even speculate.

I started to run a fever. No need for another emergency run – I was already scheduled for the clinic. I wasn't long in the chair in the infusion room before one of the nurses said, "They're going to admit you. We just have to wait for a bed." That time was hazy, but what I recall is that I felt perfectly horrible. I stayed in that chair for a very long time. I remember longing for a bed. Sleep was all I wanted.

Finally I was admitted and the tests began. I was wheeled down to Respiratory Therapy for a bronchoscopy. Someone forgot to give me the standard numbing shot to suppress the natural gag reflex. When the scope was stuck down my throat, I gagged so hard that it seemed my whole insides would come out.

After some time in the hospital, when I started to feel human and focused again, I asked Hannah, "How long have I been here?"

I was shocked when she told me "Two weeks."

"You know," I said, "I don't think I've looked in a mirror that whole time."

She responded kindly, "That's okay, Mom. You can wait a little longer."

A curious response, I thought. What I didn't know was that I had gagged with such force that I had broken all the blood vessels in and around my eyes. The sockets were ringed with black, and the whites of my eyes had turned bright red. Later, when I talked to Dot about it, she said, "Murphy, you look like a demon." I'm sure my ghastly, Halloween-appropriate appearance was very unnerving for her, Ed, Hannah, and any visitors I had.

When I was scheduled for another bronchoscopy, I knew to say to the medical personnel, "Please don't forget the Lidocaine spray." They looked at me like I was insane. "Of course we wouldn't," one said. "We *never* do a bronchoscopy without Lidocaine!" *Never*, I thought, *except when somebody forgets*.

I don't remember much of anything about those days, but at some point the diagnosis became clear: fungal pneumonia. I was put on Caspofungin, one of the worst medicines I've ever taken. I was wracked with severe chills, causing me to shake the bed violently. The extreme trembling could only be controlled with IV Demerol, about as heavy-duty a pain medication as you can find. During each infusion, I would sleep for hours.

Not being able to breathe is one of the most frightening experiences I have known. At times I coughed interminably – sometimes so severely that I feared I couldn't draw my next breath. We tried everything to stop it: cough drops, sour lemon drops, lemon juice, hot teas – anything and everything. But much of the difficulty simply had to be endured until my medications began to lessen the severity of the pneumonia. It became so clear to me then, in a way I had never before truly appreciated, how the capacity to breathe is directly related to sustaining life moment by moment.

I spent the next days and weeks suspended between worlds. I remember people coming and going. I remember somber faces. I remember that Ed was anxious, and Hannah too. Also that they were doing their dead-level best not to communicate their fears and anxieties to me.

I began talking with friends and family who were not visible to others. One afternoon Hannah invited a visitor into the room. I don't remember who she was, but no matter how cherished the friend, there were no hugs or even handshakes allowed in those days and she stood at the foot of my bed. Early in the conversation I motioned behind me and said to her, "I want you to meet our good friend Charlotta from the Southern Center for Human Rights. She's a lawyer and works against the death penalty." The visitor nodded, wished me well, and soon left.

Hannah came back from the door with a worried look on her face. "Mom, are you aware that Charlotta isn't here?"

I pulled up on my elbow, craned my neck, and looked over at the chair behind my bed. Sure enough, it was empty. I was very surprised. "Well, when did she leave?"

Hannah answered gently, "Mama, Charlotta hasn't been here today."

But I was *certain* that I had been in a conversation with Charlotta just before the other visitor arrived.

My best visit during this time was with my Dad, who had been gone from this earth for 18 months. I don't remember being "transported" – only that we were together, "over" my body on the hospital bed – over and slightly to the left. I was aware of my body below me, but I was completely undisturbed. There was a soft bright light all around us. My Dad was strong again, sitting up straight, dressed neatly in his slacks and a cheerful yellow sweater I had given him. We had a wonderful talk and were so happy to be in each other's presence. I have no idea how long it lasted, but I was sure that Dad would have called it, in his happiest tone of voice, "a good visit."

In some moments of clarity in the days that followed, I reported to Dot that I had "been with Dad." She blanched. "There was one day I came in here," she said, "and you *sounded* like Dad. It was as if his voice had inhabited you."

What was it that I experienced so dramatically? A spiritual vision? An illness-induced hallucination? Lack of oxygen to the brain? I didn't know.

What I also didn't know was just how dire my prognosis was. One day Dr. Lonial took Ed out into the hall and told him that they had done all that they could for me. The only other option was putting me on a ventilator. "But," he explained, "we don't use ventilators on the transplant floor, because people don't come off the ventilator, and we don't want to put people through that." In other words: Get ready, your wife is going to die.

Ed kept it together enough to make calls to Hannah and to Dayspring Farm in Ellijay, Georgia, where the rest of the Open Door Community was gathered for a retreat. Then, with tears coursing down his cheeks, he asked the charge nurse if there was a place he could be alone. She led him to the nurse's break room and cleared everybody out. When she left him, Ed broke down in sobs.

As it turned out, it was my turn to be a guinea pig. Amy Langston is an infectious disease specialist as well as a hematologist, and under that hat she was heading clinical trials at Emory for a drug called Posaconazole, part of a larger national study. Since I was somewhere off in LaLa Land, she asked Ed, as my medical power of attorney, if he wanted to sign papers for me to participate in the study. Given that my choices had been reduced to that or die, he did not hesitate to sign me up.

I started on the Posaconazole, and I began to get well. Palpable providence. It "just so happened" that I was a patient of Amy's, in a hospital where she was heading trials of a new life-saving drug. Without access to Posaconazole, I surely would have died of fungal pneumonia.

Nearly all the medical experts had already given me up for dead. But by some combination of providence, prayer, community, an experimental drug, and inscrutable mystery, I came through – beaten down, chewed up, looking like a dead woman walking – but alive. The choice Anthony Granberry had set before us – "faith or fear" – had indeed been a sustaining word on this long, tumultuous journey.

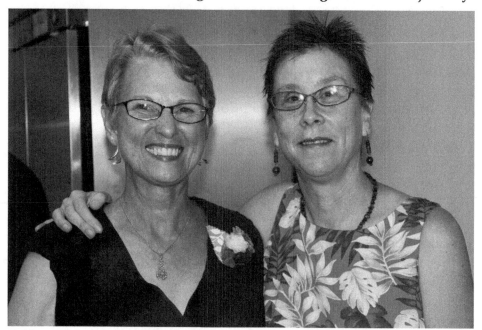

Murphy with Dr. Amelia (Amy) Langston during a healthier time, celebrating Hannah and Jason's wedding in 2012. Photo by Calvin Kimbrough

A year and a half later, in January 2006, the Open Door Community was on another week-long retreat at Dayspring Farm. I was overflowing with gratitude that I could join the rest of the community this time at this special place. Early in our life together, it had become clear that all of us at the Open Door would benefit from having somewhere to go to get breaks from our hectic and demanding urban life, and because we lived financially from a "common pot" and drew no salaries, affording vacations was difficult. Our purchase of the farm in 1987 was made possible by our friends Bill and Bonnie Neely. Bill and Ed had been classmates at Presbyterian College in the 1960s and they had helped us, through their small family foundation, to buy the 14-acre farm 88 miles north of Atlanta. Dayspring was a place of joy for us, with gardens to tend, trails to walk, and a lake for swimming nearby. We renovated the barn to provide enough sleeping space for the entire community to hold regular retreats there, and we also took individual time off and personal retreats at the farm as we could.

As we all sat in a circle in the living room of the farmhouse, Gladys spoke. She looked at me and said, "I never sit in this room now without remembering that day in August 2004 when Ed called us. The doctors had told him that you were very close to death. We were devastated. We came into this room and gathered on the floor around the coffee table. Lauren and I lighted candles. And then we prayed long and hard. We prayed and wept...wept and prayed."

Gladys had told me this before, but as she shared the story again, I heard it as if for the first time. That was the moment I suddenly knew that I had not simply had a vision, but I had indeed *been* with Dad. We had met – here, over there, or somewhere in the middle. Had he come to where I was, or had I gone to where he is? Is there some place carved out between life and death where we can, in extreme circumstances, "go?" What does it matter? It is probably not even a matter of distance. The border between "here" and "there" seemed porous – "a thin place," as they say at Iona. What I do know is that he had come to help and accompany me as I got ready to cross over.

But then, somewhere down in the place of my deepest knowing, somewhere deep down in my soul, the Spirit of God groaned within me. And the Spirit of God joined with the urgent prayers that went up from Dayspring Farm. It joined with Ed's desperate wails rising from the nurse's break room. It joined with Hannah's wracking sobs as a friend rushed her toward Emory Hospital. It joined hopes and prayers of friends and family near and far as the word spread.

And they called me back. It was as if I was on a good journey toward life in another form and realm, and the path was friendly and warm and welcoming. But my beloved ones were saying, "It is not yet time. Say goodbye to the ones over there. And come back. Your time can wait." And the Spirit sighed and said, "Yes. Return."

After so many days of descending into the depths of illness and unknowing, this was the moment I came closest to death. A critical turning point of my journey.

Hannah told me that as I was coming back to consciousness – that day, or later? – I looked at her and said excitedly, "Hannah, I've just been with Papa Tom! And he invited me to a party!" She said that she practically screamed back at me as she catapulted toward me from her chair, "Well, you tell him you can't come and you'll see him later. *Mama, you can't go with him! Not now!*"

So the party with my Dad will wait. Dad always was a very patient man. Thank you, God.

I didn't realize until the haze lifted from my brain many days after that experience how far my spirit had ventured out from my body. Even now, years later, the realization is still settling in. I was on my way – leaving those I knew and loved here – and joining another group of the beloved who had crossed over before me. But I never crossed all the way over. I am very grateful for that. But I also moved on from that moment confident that there is friendly presence and warm welcome out there waiting for me and, I expect, for us all.

My life, my destiny, my vocation, my journey have been so clearly revealed as solidarity with the human/earthly family: solidarity across every line of race, class, age, gender, and geography. Now there was the lowering of yet another boundary. I came to see my near-death experience as the ultimate gift of solidarity. Death itself does not separate us.

The passage I've loved so well in that letter of Paul's to the Roman church is, in the depth of my own experience, true: *Who will separate us from the love of Christ? Will hardship, or distress, or persecution, or famine, or nakedness, or peril, or sword?...I am convinced that neither death, nor life, nor angels, nor rulers, nor things present, nor things to come, nor powers, nor height, nor depth, nor anything else in all creation, will be able to separate us from the love of God* (Rom. 8:35, 38, NRSV).

Nothing – *nothing!* – can separate us from the love of God. Or, I would add, from each other. In the presence of God's love, we live with those who are alive, and those who have died. All of us in the human family – through all of history – united as one.

My journey with cancer became longer and more unbelievable as every year passed. Many times I walked through the halls of Winship Cancer Center and encountered one of the doctors or nurses from the hospital or clinic. If I hadn't seen them in a while, I noticed the fleeting expression on their faces that seemed to say, "I can't *believe* she's not dead yet."

Nope. As the African-American spiritual says, "Ain't Got Time to Die."

11

Transitions

When it was finally clear to my doctors that I was not going to die, I was able to go home from the hospital. In our bathroom, a "separator" connected to a long tube cranked out oxygen 24/7. I was on a long tether, so that I could go out into the wider hall outside our apartment and walk up and down to get in the "mile a day" of exercise that Dr. Langston demanded as a minimum of all her patients. After a while I was given a portable backpack with oxygen, so that Ed and I could go for a walk in Piedmont Park – and even to see a movie in a theater. I stayed on the oxygen full-time for three months and then graduated to using it only at night.

A big concern was the amount of weight I had lost in the hospital. I was skin and bones, and I needed to add some pounds for strength. This was definitely not a problem I had ever experienced before. But each week when I saw my nurse practitioner Janet Lee, she would say, "Isn't there anything you can do to eat more high-calorie foods?" These were words I *never* expected to hear from a healthcare provider.

Nelia took it as her personal duty to put the pounds on me. During those years, the Panera Bread restaurant across from Emory University generously brought by their left-over breads and pastries. Since for many of our homeless guests the Open Door meal was their only one of the day, we served high-protein, nutrient-rich foods and reserved sweets for special occasions like birthday celebrations. Now when the donations arrived, Nelia went through them, quickly wrapping up Panera's sticky nut rolls (my favorite) and other delicacies that might tempt me. Every day she made sure that I had indulged in as many yummy treats as I could take.

When I still didn't gain enough weight, Janet gently fussed at me, and Nelia took it as a personal failure. On it went through the fall. We finally learned from Amy that people with lung disease have a difficult time gaining weight because so many of the body's calories are used up simply to keep breathing. Eventually, as I healed, my weight returned to a normal level. The problem then was weaning myself off this extravagant diet!

The personal challenges of that time were aggravated by villainy on the national level. When George W. Bush was elected president that fall – despite Al Gore's winning the popular vote – despair deepened on the streets. One morning after breakfast, an angry homeless friend smashed to smithereens the huge mirror that covered the wall in the foyer of the Open Door. It was a great loss. We had often noticed that people who came in off the streets bedraggled and beaten down stopped in front of the mirror on their way out after a shower and a visit to our clothes closet. The men would straighten their shirts, the women would put finishing touches on their hair, and all would raise their heads and walk out the door just a little taller.

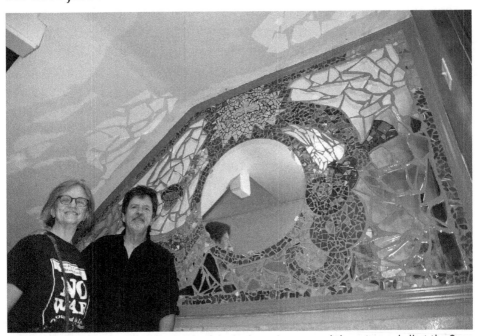

Nelia Kimbrough's design from the shards of the broken mirror graced the entrance hall at the Open Door. Bruce Bishop, a member of the extended community, visited to help put finishing touches on the mosaic. Photo by Calvin Kimbrough

Nelia gathered up all the shattered pieces. She also began to save the shards of every plate that broke in the community. With our faithful artist friend Bruce Bishop, she used these to create a mosaic, depicting two hands holding a piece of broken bread and a chalice being poured out. It was a stunning symbol of the restoration that can emerge out of brokenness, a beautiful example of Nelia's "found object" art pieces that would grace our life in the years to come. We gave it a place of honor – in the space where the mirror had once hung.

It took a long time to get the fungal pneumonia under control and, when it was, I was back on track toward a bone marrow transplant. Once again my friends and family rallied around, determined to find a matching donor. Exactly 10 years after my first death sentence, as my 57th birthday loomed in March 2005, some 300 friends filled the sanctuary at Covenant Presbyterian Church in downtown Atlanta for an "Ain't Got Time to Die" concert and party. The gala affair was organized by Collin Lines, a friend and member of Covenant Presbyterian; Margaret Randolph, a physical therapist (who graciously brought her massage table to the Open Door from time to time to care for my weary body); Ray Quinnely, who delighted us throughout my many recoveries with her gifts of delicious homemade sorbet; Millie Deanes, a Montessori teacher who cooked rice and beans at the Open Door every Friday night from 1982 until 2015; Elise Witt, a professional musician who always kept our hearts alive and our spirits up as she sat on the edge of my bed at home or in the hospital and sang; and my ever-faithful friend, Mary Sinclair.

The goal of the evening was to recruit more potential bone marrow donors and to raise money to pay for those who wanted to enroll in the registry but couldn't afford the fee. The spirited Joyce and Jackie, a well-known vocal duo, performed folk and civil rights favorites and some of their original songs. Just Voices, a fabulous *a capella* choir directed by Liz Frazier, sang at the front of the church to the throng while people took turns going to the back to sign up with the bone marrow registry. At the end of the concert, Liz invited everybody who had ever sung "Ain't Got Time to Die" with a choral group to come and join Just Voices and Joyce and Jackie in a rousing final number. It was unforgettable – they truly "raised the roof" of Covenant's sanctuary!

It was a great party, but despite this generous, loving effort, no match was found among the crowd for me. And as the months rolled by, it became clear that – though the transplant foundation had searched all over the country and even expanded into the international registry to try to find a match – there was none to be found. This prompted more jokes among my friends about the lengths to which I go to be *different*. I was extremely relieved when a CAT scan in the fall of 2006 showed that the chemotherapy had driven the lymphoma back into remission, so the bone marrow transplant could be set aside.

Though the fungal pneumonia was always with me, the next years brought periods of relatively good health, with a few crises interspersed. Gradually I was able to take baby steps toward taking up more normal activity. I was glad to get back to the prisons and to visit with our homeless friends as they came and went. But my doctors discouraged me from serving in the biweekly free medical and foot clinics that we hosted at the Open Door and from helping with the soup kitchen. I remained in a vulnerable state, and they didn't want me to catch a random germ that could make me very sick again. In spite of these limitations and a vastly increased need for rest, I found that being upright was a joy, and being able to have more time with friends and co-workers was a delight. I was overwhelmed with gratitude.

In September 2008, a routine CAT scan raised concern about cancerous lesions on my spleen. But a follow-up PET scan showed that the small bumps were not cancer after all – prompting a childhood friend to write and tell me that I should have taken care of those pimples on my spleen long ago. But the radiologist did identify several malignant nodes in my chest, between my lungs. This was not what we wanted to hear.

My cancer had morphed into an "indolent" lymphoma – so named because it is very slow-growing. Even my cancer had become lazy! Our dear friend Lewis Sinclair, who died in 2008 at the age of 93, fought indolent lymphoma for almost 20 years. When he was diagnosed in the early 1990s, he said dryly, "Well, what else do you expect a lazy old man to have?"

There were a few treatment options to ponder. Because the cancer was growing so slowly, there was no need to rush the decision. I wanted to consider it carefully with my doctors – and, of course, with Hannah Loring-Davis, RN!

After her time working with *The Other Side* magazine in Philadelphia, Hannah had returned to Atlanta in 2003. She attended massage therapy school and volunteered to be the coordinator of our weekly Open Door foot clinic. Homelessness is particularly damaging to feet, and people flocked to the clinic to receive care for blisters, bruises, and callouses that resulted from spending so much time on their feet – often in ill-fitting shoes, or without socks, facing the constant danger of frostbite during the cold months.

During my first week in the hospital in 2004, Hannah came into my room one afternoon and said, "I've been thinking, and I realize that I'm happiest when I'm working with my patients in the foot clinic on Wednesday evenings. I'm going to nursing school." She had been strictly a Humanities student in college, and her announcement caught Ed and me by surprise. But soon we thought, *Well, of course!* Hannah has been providing a form of nursing care to me ever since she was daily cleaning my gaping surgical wound as a tenth-grader.

When she got close to graduation from nursing school in Atlanta, Hannah decided that the one job she most wanted was in the Surgical Intensive Care Unit at Johns Hopkins Hospital in Baltimore. She applied, interviewed a week later, and was offered a position on the spot. She cared for people coming out of surgery, many of them from kidney, liver, and other transplants. These didn't always turn out well, and Hannah was often the person who had to talk with family members when a patient was dying or close to death. She had to wade into difficult conversations about when to stop treatment, or unhook machines, and let a loved one go. Most of the families were totally unprepared to make such weighty decisions, and Hannah was a compassionate and sensitive presence with people facing the greatest crises of their lives.

She seemed so young to be doing this challenging work. But the truth is that Hannah has been personally grappling with the reality of death since my first diagnosis, when she was 15. And she was raised with a daily, intimate awareness of suffering and death, which resided right alongside the joy of our life. As a result, she has an unusual level of maturity and capacity to talk about death without coming apart at the seams. She has a gift for working with patients and families staring death in the face.

After six years working in the Surgical ICU, Hannah pursued a clinical nursing specialty in end-of-life care and earned her Master's degree from Johns Hopkins. She taught for six years in the School of Nursing at Notre Dame of Maryland University, and was then recruited to teach at the School of Nursing at the University of Maryland in downtown Baltimore, where she is now. She is also nearing the end of a Ph.D. program through Catholic University, focused on hospice care in prisons.

A great gift along the way of Hannah's journey has been Amy Langston's support and encouragement. It's been wonderful how Amy has included Hannah in the conversations about my care and listened carefully to her questions and concerns. Occasionally Hannah calls her with a question from her work, and Amy takes the time to explain things to her, using medical terminology that Hannah understands. I think Hannah takes a little pride in the fact that she can have conversations with Amy that we can't comprehend! It's a beautiful thing.

My first choice for treatment was participation in another clinical trial on a new drug under Amy's supervision. For 13 years I had been the recipient of many new drugs and protocols tested by others, and I was glad when I had been able to participate in the clinical trial on Posaconazole – which benefitted not only me but many others – and I was anxious to be helpful again. A second option was outpatient chemotherapy. And the third was a regimen involving infusions of the immunotherapy drug Rituxan and a new drug called Bexxar, combined with a radioactive element to blast the lymphoma cells – more harsh than the chemo.

I was awaiting a lumbar puncture that would help determine which course to follow, when we got word that Jack Alderman had been given an execution date of September 16th. Ed and I had known Jack for 30 of his 34 years on death row. He was one of the last of the "old-timers" we had gotten to know so many years ago when we began our work on the row.

Even with all the restrictions of death row, Jack had fashioned a life that he could call good. He was a very thoughtful human being and a father figure to many younger men on death row. He wrote letters for those who could not read and write. Jack always maintained his innocence of the crime of which he was convicted, and he had done the hard work of releasing his initial bitterness toward the man who most certainly did commit the murder, and whose testimony was the only evidence against him.

We sat with Jack and other friends during the days leading up to his appointment with the lethal needle. Jack walked through the death watch as he had walked through the three decades we had known him: with composure and dignity. During those final hours together, we reminisced, told stories, laughed, cried, hugged, and provided as much comfort for each other as possible in such an awful situation. They killed Jack Alderman right on schedule. But his final days and weeks were spent in gratitude for the life he had lived.

We had barely caught our breath when we got word that Troy Davis had been handed an execution date. This had happened a few times before, and each time he had received a stay. But we knew that one day he would not, and so every time we had to prepare for the worst. When I got the news, I felt like I had been run over by a Mack truck.

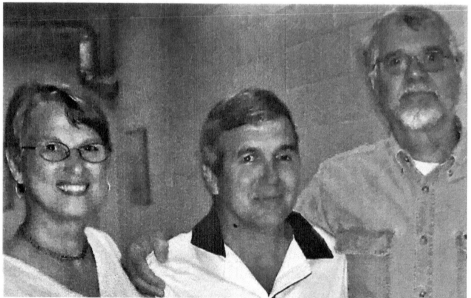

Jack Alderman in the prison visiting room with Murphy and Ed on the day before his execution. Photo by Wesley Baker, prison staff

Ed and I were scheduled to go to Los Angeles for the annual Catholic Worker retreat there. I struggled with being away during Troy's execution. But due to a widespread – even global – belief in Troy's innocence, people from literally all over the world were supporting him. Groups such as Amnesty International and the NAACP, as well as individuals from President Jimmy Carter to Archbishop Desmond Tutu, advocated on his behalf. But probably more to the point, I simply didn't feel that I could take another execution less than a week after Jack's.

From Los Angeles, Ed and I stayed in touch with Troy's sister Martina and learned, to our great relief, that he was granted another stay. The state ultimately took his life three years later, on September 21, 2011. At his funeral, Martina was in a wheelchair, severely weakened by breast cancer. She had been a tireless advocate for her brother, persistently proclaiming his innocence and working for his release. I believe it was an act of pure will, taking all of her strength, to stay alive to see Troy through. She died soon after her beloved brother did.

Jack's execution had been a huge blow, and Troy's showed once again just how wrongheaded the system of capital punishment is. Ed and I began to feel at that time that it was the end of an era in our ministry on death row.

The nodes in my chest were too close to my lungs to risk a biopsy, which would have been required for the clinical trial or the Bexxar regimen. Amy ordered a chemotherapy protocol called Gemcitabine Navelbine ("Gem-Nav"), telling me that, after all the chemo I'd been through, this six-month course would be "a walk in the park." After I endured a few tough weeks on it, my nephew Todd Moye, a civil rights historian, wondered if Amy had meant the Kelly Ingram Park in Birmingham, Alabama. I'm well aware, as is Todd, of the dangers of comparing anything I've experienced to the horror of African-American marchers, including children, being attacked by police dogs and blasted by fire hoses in the 1963 Birmingham Campaign. But he did have a point: Gemcitabine Navelbine was unlike any park I've walked through. Amy had a valid point though, too: it was significantly easier than my previous experiences of chemotherapy.

Knowing that I was going to lose my hair again, I had a particular concern about two young children who had become quite precious to me. Visiting them at the end of September, I did not want them to be shocked to see me bald when I visited the next time. It seemed the best thing to do was invite them to help me pre-emptively lose my hair. "For *real*?!" they exclaimed in unison when I explained what we were going to do.

They took turns cutting big chunks of my hair and watching them fall to the kitchen floor. At 4 and 6 years old, they had a hard time accepting that what they were doing wasn't naughty, but they got into it, giggling at points but also taking their task very seriously.

Then their mother took clippers and shaped what was left into a crewcut, and we all laughed hilariously. Their father, who regularly shaved his own head, lathered me up and took it all away with a razor.

When it was over, the 4-year-old just kept staring at me and saying "Wow!" over and over. The 6-year-old gazed thoughtfully at my bald, shiny noggin and said, "Hmmm...I think I like it better *with* hair." Ed leaned against the kitchen wall and quietly wept.

In October we celebrated the Festival of Shelters, as we did every year at the Open Door. Rooted in the Jewish tradition of Sukkoth, a harvest festival that calls to mind the temporary booths the Israelites lived in during their time in the wilderness after the Exodus from slavery (Ex. 23:16; Lev. 23:34), its liturgy seems made for homeless people. We began by spending a night in Woodruff Park in downtown Atlanta with our homeless friends, and in later years in the front yard at 910 Ponce de Leon.

Nelia always brought her extraordinary creativity to our communal construction of a *sukkah*, weaving twigs around limbs for the sides, leaving gaps in the roof open to the sky as a reminder of our vulnerability. She and Gladys handed out blank cardboard stars to everyone in the yard and to people who came to the soup kitchen, asking them to write what gives them hope. We hung the stars from the twigs of the ceiling, so that the hopes of the homeless sheltered and covered us.

Each evening of the festival ended with a feast. I was enjoying a piece of fried chicken when the gut-wrenching pain hit. Next thing I knew, I was at the hospital getting my gall bladder removed. All I remember about that surgery, which seemed so minor compared to everything else I'd been through, was coming to in a groggy state and hearing a nurse say, "She needs the Lawdy." I wondered how she knew. Yes, I did indeed need "the Lawdy," a common Southern folk term for "the Lord." I guess I laughed when I realized that she was actually assessing my pain level and declaring, "She needs Dilaudid." I still need the Lawdy, but I'm glad the nurse recognized that in that moment I needed a good wallop of pain medication, too!

Once I was fully recovered, I resumed chemotherapy, but there seemed to be no end of things that could go wrong. By the spring of 2010, I was diagnosed with hypogammaglobulinemia (I still have to practice pronouncing it). Basically, my immune system was shot. I began having infusions of intravenous immune globulin (IVIG), extracted from 60 units of donated blood, every four to six weeks. I remember sitting in the infusion chair one day thinking, "It's like I'm going to the library every few weeks, checking out a new immune system." I became concerned that I was using up far more than my share of available medical resources. I felt a little better when it was explained to me that other patients got the platelets and other elements of those 60 pints of blood.

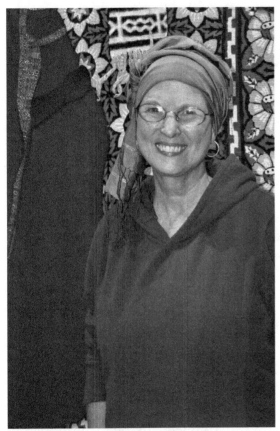

Friends sent many beautiful scarves and head coverings during chemo times, including this especially loved one from a women's cooperative in Thailand, courtesy of Marie Fortune. Photo by Calvin Kimbrough

Just when I thought I was going to get through this course of chemotherapy without an actual hospitalization (something you should never voice out loud), the shingles struck. I had suffered this annoying scourge before, but this time was different. Usually shingles attack only one side of the body, stopped at the spine from crossing over. But not mine. "I've never seen this happen to anybody else," the doctor told me.

Boy, was I tired of hearing those words. How many times had it been? I just wanted to be normal.

"We're going to admit you," the doctor said.

"For *shingles*?"

The danger of shingles on both sides, I was told, is that the next step in the progression of the virus is to the brain or liver. So off to a hospital bed I went for several days of IV Acyclovir, a wonder drug that saved me from the furious pain and mind-wrecking itch that visited me with previous bouts of shingles. I was in isolation, which meant that all my caregivers had to wear paper gowns, masks, and gloves to come in. One pregnant resident talked with me only through the cracked door. After I left the hospital with a prescription for Acyclovir pills, I asked Amy how long I would have to take it. "Forever," she said. And so another drug was added to my daily apothecary.

During chemotherapy, my doctors had requested that I not travel farther than half an hour away. When I finished, Ed and I decided we needed to celebrate the end of another long period of months chained to Emory University Hospital. We made an autumn journey through the Appalachian Mountains, all the way up the Blue Ridge Parkway to the Skyline Drive. At the northern end, we spent a week with Hannah in her row house in Baltimore's Patterson Park neighborhood. As always, we had great fun. And this time we met her new boyfriend, Jason Buc, a firefighter and paramedic in Howard County, Maryland.

It was a journey of glorious restoration. As Ed and I headed back toward home on the Skyline Drive, a chilly fall rain settled over the darkening forest. Somewhere around Big Meadows in Virginia's

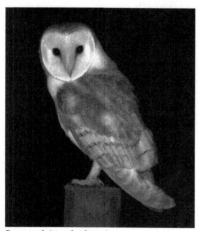

Barn owl (stock photo)

Shenandoah National Park the rain stopped, but everything was wet and shiny in our headlights, and fallen yellow leaves decorated the road's black surface. We came around a curve in the deep darkness and stopped abruptly for a large bird standing in the middle of the road. The creature was a barn owl. It swiveled its head without the slightest movement in the rest of its great body and stared straight at us. Then it lifted its enormous wings and flew up and away.

A chill ran down my spine, and I was certain that this had been a special visitation. Later I learned that in Native American legends, the owl – and in particular the barn owl – often symbolizes death. But the owl is also seen as a spirit creature associated with wisdom, and is sometimes believed to indicate the coming of an important transition.

I have remembered that mystical encounter with gratitude. It came at a time when I was moving past treatment into another period of health. I had just finished my fifth regimen of chemotherapy and, once again, I had survived. I keep a picture of the full face of a barn owl in my prayer book, and I am thankful to this particular beautiful creature at home in the Shenandoah National Park for the gift bestowed.

My September PET scan that year was not so good. Some of the malignant nodes in my chest had shrunk, but some had grown. After enduring chemo, you really don't want to hear that any of the cancer cells are growing. Amy and my physician's assistant, Somi King, declared it a draw – stable, more or less – and that was good enough to go on for the moment.

I had to return for another PET scan in the spring. I was braced for bad news. Hannah was as well, and she and Jason flew down from Baltimore to be present for my clinic appointment. Somi – with all her gentleness and humor – went through the preliminaries with us. She checked me up and down, listened to my lungs, told us about her children.

Then Amy came in. Wasting no time after hugs all around, she shrugged her shoulders, grinned, and said, "I can't account for this, but everything has shrunk." It took a minute for my brain to make the shift. *Shrunk?!* Even those rogue nodes that were growing after six months of chemo? Yes. That's what she said.

We were overwhelmed with joy. Once more the trajectory of my cancer had defied lymphoma's logic. The beast had backed up again. I don't remember what we said or did after that – just the joy.

And the "But…"

While the scan brought nothing but good news about the lymphoma, there was a new place "of concern": a small area of "hypermetabolic activity" in my left breast. The radiologist recommended follow-up with my primary care doctor and a mammogram. I was so overjoyed about the lymphoma that this barely registered, and we all parted on a very happy note. Though it was the first week of Lent, it felt like Mardi Gras was still in full force. *"Laissez les bon temps rouler!"* Let the good times roll, indeed!

Lent proceeded. On Good Friday I felt up to performing my first-person telling of the Passion story, a dramatic presentation that I had offered in years past. It meant so much to me to be back in action. Over the years the power of the story has grown in me: the overlay of fighting against and waiting for the execution of our friends on death row and the story of the arrest, torture, trial, and execution of Jesus the Jew. The experience and the story have come together and live in my bones.

Easter morning found me with my community in the front yard – not standing at a distance on the second floor porch as I had the year before and on several other Easter Sundays. Once again Resurrection felt like a personal, lived experience.

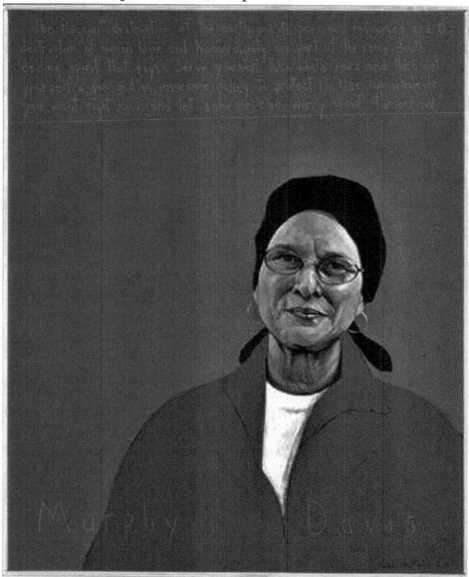

During Murphy's treatment in 2010, Rob Shetterly visited and painted this portrait of her for his series Americans Who Tell the Truth (www.americanswhotellthetruth.org).

I returned to Grady for my first visit with my new primary care doctor. I had not been a patient in the grand old hospital for seven years, and I was surprised to realize how happy I was to be back, feeling very much "at home" with staff and companions in the waiting room. I spent an hour with the diminutive, brilliant, and compassionate Dr. Jada Bussey-Jones.

She could not find a lump in my left breast. "If something is there," she assured me, "it's really small and really early." I left with a referral for a mammogram in hand. The woman in Central Scheduling asked, "Can you come back for this tomorrow?"

Tomorrow?! "Did you say *tomorrow*?" I said. "I thought I was at Grady!" She chuckled and set up the appointment.

The lump was barely visible but, sure enough, there it was on the mammogram. And why wouldn't it be? We diagnose cancer with an array of procedures – X-rays, CAT scans, PET scans – all pumping radioactivity into the body. We treat it with the toxic poison of chemotherapy and more doses of radiation. Why should it be a surprise that cancer begins to show up in other places?

The interventional radiologist moved me across the hall for a sonogram. "It's clearly very small," she declared, "but we need to schedule you quickly for a stereotactic biopsy." The biopsy was on May 25th, Ed's and my 36th wedding anniversary. All I will say about it is that this grueling procedure was definitely not part of letting the good times roll. Two and a half hours later, I left with an appointment to return on June 3rd.

That day Dr. Joel Okoli burst into the examining room with an entourage of staff: a surgical fellow, a resident, a research nurse, the regular clinic nurse, and two Morehouse medical students. Bad news, good news. It *was* cancer; but it was small, early, and not very aggressive.

We discussed my bizarre medical history. "Clearly God has work for you to do yet," the doctor declared in his East African brogue, "and we will pray for this to be only a small event in your journey so that you may continue to do God's work." We laughed raucously while speaking of some of the absurdities of this journey. Ed said later that the medical students were standing in slack-jawed amazement. Maybe they hadn't before encountered a patient receiving a cancer diagnosis like it was just another pesky insect.

Dr. Okoli told us with great excitement and exquisite detail about the time he had breakfast with Dr. Denis Burkitt during a medical conference. While everyone around them enjoyed bacon and eggs, the doctor famous for discovering the link between lack of dietary fiber and cancer ate dry, rather tasteless, high-fiber cereal – and Dr. Okoli felt compelled to join him.

I liked Dr. Okoli very much and regretted having to tell him that I would likely need to have my breast-cancer care at Emory's Winship Cancer Center, for the sake of continuity. "Well," Dr. Okoli said in parting, "whether your care is with us or not, I will pray for you." Grace abounds: unearned blessing, unexpected laughter, unanticipated joy.

I called Amy Langston on the way home. I was already scheduled to see her the following Monday morning and she invited me to come in early. "I need some time with you," she said. "Come to the clinic early and we'll discuss it. Oh, Murphy, I'm so sorry." Amy loves us. She not only "provides care," she cares. Again and again we realize the promise "I will never put on you more than you can bear." Before we ever have to contemplate bearing a heavier load, the shoulders of good souls are moving forward to bear it with us.

On Sunday night I called Bill Eley. Bill, beloved teacher and associate dean of Emory Medical School, has spent his adult life as a medical oncologist fighting breast cancer, researching racial and class disparities in detection, treatment, and outcomes, and staunchly advocating for Grady Hospital. I have known him since 2002, when he suddenly appeared in my hospital room with several medical students and said, "Hey, Murphy! Would you talk to these students about what you're going through and what it's like to be a patient here?" We were friends immediately.

Now Ed and I were very glad we could turn to one we already loved and respected. "Oh no!" Bill lamented. "Of course we'll get you into the clinic as quickly as we can. Now, Murphy, you know you're going get through this just like you've gotten through all the rest..."

Bright and early Monday morning, Amy was concerned but encouraging. She was glad I was going to see Bill and told me about the two highly respected breast surgeons at Winship. It was decided that I would see Sheryl Gabram. On Wednesday Bill spent two hours with us. We talked about lots of mutual interests and friends. We met some of the other staff, and Ed and I struggled to absorb another truckload of new information.

We left with an appointment for the following Wednesday with Dr. Gabram. Bill assured us: "When you've seen the surgery team, Amy and Sheryl and I will sit down together in the same room to consider all the aspects of your medical history and status and make the best recommendations we can."

How is it that we are so blessed? How could it be that I – a "charity case" – could be the recipient of some of the best medical care the world has to offer? How could it be that we – who gave up salaries, savings, and health insurance 30 years ago – are recipients of such lavish grace?

Dr. Sheryl Gabram was warm and welcoming in the surgery clinic. Clearly Bill and Amy had talked with her. Once again the way had been prepared, and I felt at ease and sure with her. She explained the "oncoplastic reduction" she would perform: a lumpectomy, removing the tumor with very wide margins and a lymph node, then testing it to see whether she needed to remove more nodes. When she finished, a plastic surgeon would come in to remove the same amount of tissue from the other breast, leaving me with smaller and balanced breasts. "Perky," Dr. Loskin promised later in his office. Perky breasts – just what an old woman is looking for!

I was very clear about one thing. "No more radiation," I told Amy. It had become a sort of mantra with me. "Given my lymphoma," I explained, "I don't think I'll live long enough to die of breast cancer anyway."

Amy understood, but the radiation oncologist had to sign off on it. Young Dr. Mylin Torres turned out to be a friend of one of our cherished anti-death penalty lawyers, so we felt an easy rapport with her and a definite hope that my wish would be granted. A panel of gurus had to make the final decision. When the surgery was scheduled, I thought, *Wow, no mention of radiation. I sure must have been convincing.*

A month later when we saw Amy again, we learned that she had put her foot down hard with the others: "No way you're going to radiate her. Forget it." I doubt if anyone dared to argue after that. "Well, of course," she explained to us. "You're already at very high risk for leukemia with all the treatment you've had. I wasn't going to let anybody add more radiation to that risk." That came as news to me.

The surgery proceeded, Ed at my side, my community and friends praying their hearts out, Hannah flying down from Baltimore to help me recuperate. It was not half as bad as we had expected – perhaps because, even though it was my fourth major surgery, it was the first I experienced without having to go right into chemotherapy. After two pretty intense weeks, I began to feel better and stronger by the day. Within a month I was swimming and hiking again.

All pathology reports were good, so no follow-up therapy was recommended. Bill Eley said, "Maybe it sounds odd to say we're not going to do anything more for you but take the best care of you we can." Four weeks after the surgery, Bill and I joined Dr. Mary Dolan for a session with second-year Emory medical students on breast cancer. "I want them to understand," said Bill, "that disease doesn't always move like you learned it in a textbook."

Well, yes," I said, "then I would be your specimen." A number of the students were contributing their time and skill to the Open Door's weekly Harriett Tubman Free Clinic, and the time with them was great fun, with lots of questions and lots of laughs. It seemed that I could set aside the threat of breast cancer.

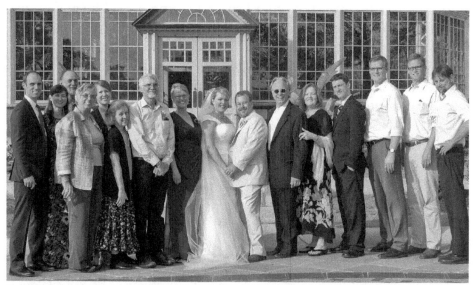

Murphy's family gathered for Hannah and Jason's wedding in Baltimore in May 2012. Left to right: James and Emily Davis, Mac Davis, Dorothy (Dot) Davis Moye, Sarah Moye, Tracy Smith, Ed and Murphy, Hannah and Jason, Robin and Linda Williams, Alex Davis-Smith, Will Moye, Todd Moye, Les Davis. Photo by Alison Reader, Framing Faces

On May 12th, 2012, Hannah and Jason got married. The evening before, Jason and his brothers barbecued and grilled chicken for the rehearsal dinner, a picnic on a hill overlooking the Chesapeake Bay with a throng of friends. The service was held in Brown Memorial

Park Avenue Presbyterian Church in Baltimore, with Revs. Andrew Foster-Connors and Lauren (now Cogswell Ramseur) officiating. A gaggle of Hannah's friends from Guilford College played bluegrass music before the service. Robin and Linda Williams, well known to fans of *A Prairie Home Companion,* sang – Robin is my first cousin.

Afterward, guests were enjoying a beautiful wedding reception with an elegant buffet among the tropical flowers and trees at the Baltimore City Conservatory and Botanic Gardens – when a piercing and persistent fire alarm went off. Before long, the shrill, blaring sirens of fire trucks were added to the mix, as several raced up and stopped out front. Assuming that Hannah had arranged a surprise arrival of his firefighting buddies, Jason looked at her and said, "What have you done?"

Hannah, who hardly would have chosen to interrupt her wedding reception in this manner, said, "I don't know anything about this." It was clear that she was telling the truth when they noticed that the fire trucks were from the Baltimore City Fire Department. It turned out that the caterer had overheated something in the oven, setting off the alarm. The firefighters capitalized on the moment, posing good-naturedly for pictures with the bride and groom, allowing the wedding couple to brandish their axes and fire hoses.

In August, I met up with Joyce Hollyday at Lake Santeetlah in western North Carolina, a beautiful spot surrounded by the Nantahala National Forest. My dear friends Marie Fortune and Anne Ganley have a cabin at the edge of the lake that has been in Marie's family for years. Anne is a psychologist who has worked to reduce male violence, and Marie is renowned in church circles for her work against clergy sexual abuse and domestic violence. Their cabin was a perfect place to spend six weeks of focused time to make some progress on this memoir.

Joyce showed up with a key lime pie, one of my favorites. I knew by then that I was allergic to dairy products and, sadly, had to give up several things I especially enjoyed, with key lime pie being high on the list. Joyce had found a recipe for the pie made with silken tofu instead of sweetened condensed milk. It was a thoughtful gesture, but even she admitted with a laugh that this little experiment left something to be desired (although it was far better, she said, than her attempt to make gluten-free baklava for a friend with celiac disease using Asian rice-paper wrappers instead of phyllo dough).

CHAPTER 11

Joyce and I worked hard – discussing, outlining, writing, editing, rewriting. But we also enjoyed daily swims in the lake, sunset sips of wine on the rocking-chair porch of nearby Snowbird Mountain Lodge, and an unforgettable meal of fresh mountain trout in a local restaurant. Grateful for a wonderful time together and for the work we accomplished, we parted with a strong sense of momentum on the book and a pile of tasks to tackle to move it forward. I was feeling good.

So it was a bit of a shock when I discovered shortly after I returned home that the breast cancer was back. Just 15 months after Amy had advocated so strongly against my getting more radiation, I was back to it. A visit to the dermatologist had led to the biopsy of a small "pimple" on my left breast. "Strange...*very* strange," mused Dr. Gabram. I seemed unable to achieve anything resembling a "normal" medical condition. I had a simple outpatient lumpectomy followed by six weeks of radiation. It was clear, given what Amy had said about my high risk for leukemia, that she felt that radiation was the only way to save my life.

So I felt awful all over again. And my writing had to be shelved for a while, as it would be many more times before this memoir was completed. If I had had any idea that it would take almost two decades to write, with multiple health interruptions, I might never have waded into it. I'm grateful for the strong encouragement of many friends and family who kept me at it, anticipating that someday there actually would *be* a book. Standing out among them were Julie Martin and Anne Wheeler, who offered not only personal encouragement but also administrative support, Ed and Hannah, Mary Sinclair, Nelia Kimbrough, and Marie Fortune, who never wavered on the conviction that I must finish the work.

On July 28th, 2013, the Open Door Community was just finishing up another retreat at Dayspring Farm, when our long-time member Ralph Dukes became quite ill. Ralph, a lifelong smoker and alcoholic, had come to live with us from a rough 30 years on the streets. He stayed sober for all the years he was among us – and he was always the first one up, well before dawn, to make the coffee on the early mornings that we served breakfast at Butler Street C.M.E. Church.

At Dayspring Ralph's long struggle with emphysema caught up with him and we had to take him to the small Gilmer County

132

Hospital. A few days later, Ed, Dick, and I drove him the 88 miles back to a nursing care center on Auburn Avenue in Atlanta, to receive the round-the-clock care he needed. The process of getting him admitted was complicated and exhausting, but Ed and I – who were counting on a week of personal time at Dayspring after the community retreat ended – decided to go ahead and drive back that night.

We arrived soon after midnight and sat on the porch for a while, debriefing the day. About 1:30 we went inside and discovered a voicemail message on the phone. "I hope you're doing well," the weak and muffled voice said. "I'm not. I need you all to come."

We immediately got back in the car and made it to Mike and Amy Vosburg-Casey's home in Atlanta about 3 o'clock in the morning. Mike was clearly coming to the end of a two-year struggle with colon cancer. Though he was a "cradle Catholic," he wanted Ed and me to be his pastors for the transition, and we were honored by his request.

Hannah flew down from Baltimore the next day, and she and Mike's brother Dan lovingly tended to him, as they had to me when I had fainted at Mike and Amy's wedding. Hannah was pregnant, awaiting a birth as she midwifed a death. Michael Edwin Vosburg-Casey died on July 31st, surrounded by love and grief and thanksgiving for this wonderful, quirky, committed man. Just 39 years old, he was a great soul lost far too early. It was particularly sad that his precious, then-3-year-old daughter Elena would miss out on growing up with such an extraordinary father. We held his funeral in the backyard of the Open Door.

Hannah gave birth four months later, on December 4th, 2013. Ed and I were with her in Baltimore for the wonderful event. She had to have a C-section and was still a bit drugged and groggy when she looked up, babe in arms, and said to me, "Mama, it's Michaela." She and Jason had named their daughter in honor of our beloved Mike. I still remember how awestruck Jason was as he held her. That adoration has continued – and become mutual between father and daughter – and Ed and I are grateful to have a son-in-law who is such a devoted father.

I thought back to almost 20 years earlier, when I had prayed with every ounce of my strength to live long enough to see Hannah graduate from high school. After a time my prayer shifted to a hope to see her graduate from college. And then to be with her through her wedding. I could barely fathom the miracle of being present as she gave birth to our precious granddaughter.

The barn owl stares out from my prayer book and reminds me every day that death is inevitable. But so is life. The circle is never-ending. Thanks be to God, who continues – despite it all – to breathe astonishing new life into the world.

12

Dislocation

Ed and I always assumed that we would live out our days at the Open Door in Atlanta. We never imagined that it would all end. In June 2016 we sent a letter to our supporters that began, "This is a letter we never thought we would have to write, and it's breaking our hearts. We have come to a time that the Open Door Community cannot move forward in the way that we have lived and worked for the past 35 years."

Several realities prompted this agonizing decision. The six of us elder leaders of the community – Dick and Gladys Rustay, Nelia and Calvin Kimbrough, Ed and I – were facing a variety of illnesses and the physical challenges of aging. We simply could no longer sustain the pace and the demand. We had hoped to turn over the ministry reins to younger folks who would carry on the vision, and we mentored several over the years with this intent. But none stepped forward to take up committed, long-term leadership of the Open Door and its outreach.

Over the years we watched our neighborhood change before our eyes. When we moved into it in 1981, it was rundown, dotted with abandoned buildings. Its often violent streets were filled with homeless people and prostitutes. But – replicating the trend in most U.S. cities – our inner-city neighborhood was becoming more gentrified every year, as people of wealth streamed in to be closer to the conveniences the city offers.

On our block, high-rises housing the poor were transformed into upscale condos; personal care homes for people suffering with mental illnesses were changed into professional offices; mom-and-pop diners were torn down and replaced with fancy white-tablecloth restaurants. And homeless people were being pushed farther and farther away. Our beloved neighborhood, we realized with great anguish, had become an unbearably inhospitable space for the poor.

As tens of millions of dollars poured into the buildings around us, we were increasingly aware that we could no longer afford to maintain our massive, 100-year-old home. In the previous two years alone, we had spent tens of thousands of dollars to replace its roof, repair and renovate the heavily used shower room, replace the aged sewer pipes, and fix the drainage problems that turned our basement into a lake with every heavy rain – a result of the extra run-off from all the new construction and paving around us, which simply overwhelmed our ancient plumbing.

The decision to close was excruciating. But we knew it was necessary. Though we found it hard for a while to see anything positive in it, Ed and I ultimately came to understand the change as a gift. Our choice to create community with the homeless poor – to live in the same space where we served hundreds of people each week – had meant that the stress was relentless, and those of us in leadership rarely got a break. The needs never stopped. There was always another knock on the door. Our home was a soup kitchen, a medical clinic, a storefront church, a crisis response center. Creating community with people off the streets and out of prison made the Open Door distinct and brought unique blessings – but they came at a high price.

Ed and I identified a deep longing within us to live simply in a smaller space. Slowly, we and the others began to embrace new plans for our lives. We all decided to live closer to family – Dick and Gladys in Vancouver, Washington, and Nelia and Calvin in Nashville, Tennessee. Hannah told us that she and Jason always assumed that they would take care of Ed and me when we couldn't take care of ourselves. She encouraged us to join them in Baltimore while we were "still on our feet." Then, she reasoned, when the time came that we needed a higher level of care, we would already be in place. Being close-by grandparents to Michaela, who was an energetic and curious 2-year-old by then, was no small incentive for our choice to take Hannah up on her plan.

We six Open Door elders were on a roller coaster of emotions, looking forward with anticipation to new things while tearfully lamenting the demise of the life we had known for so long. What felt overwhelming at times was our grief about leaving our friends in

Georgia prisons and the formerly homeless ones with whom we had shared life for so many years – and our fear that they would feel abandoned. We helped a few of the latter find work and places to live. We located space for about a dozen in personal care and nursing homes around Atlanta. We were grateful that one of our longtime friends – an alcoholic with an intellectual disability resulting from childhood encephalitis, who had stayed sober at the Open Door for 13 years – was taken in by his sister. Sadly, we later learned that he had stayed with her only three days and was back living on the streets.

We began the arduous process of selling and closing down our large property on Ponce de Leon Avenue and Dayspring Farm. Our dear friend Martin Lehfeldt directed us to Ben White, an attorney with a renowned Atlanta law firm and an expert on non-profit law. He generously worked pro bono to guide us through dissolving the Open Door as it was.

We felt the agony of knowing that our property was prime real estate, grieving the apparent inevitability that anyone who could afford the three-million-dollar appraisal price would turn it into one more falling domino in the gentrification scheme. We worked hard with ministry colleagues and a Jewish synagogue on an alternative, seizing momentary glimpses of hope that our former home would be spared demolition and that some type of human service would continue in it.

But those hopes quickly evaporated. Although the Presbytery of Greater Atlanta had not contributed to any oversight, maintenance, or improvements on the building in 35 years – or participated in the ministry that went on there – it was still half owner of the property and commandeered the sale. Through a process of committees and closed bids to which we had no access, Presbytery officials sold our home to a big-time developer. After costs, the real estate agent's sizable commission, and the Presbytery's claim on half of the profit, we ended up with far less than we had anticipated.

Making the transition to living on our own felt like a huge leap. We had, many years earlier, sold our family homes and emptied our personal savings accounts. We had drawn no salaries at the Open Door and had no IRAs or 401(k) retirement plans. But we three couples are able to live simply on small monthly stipends drawn from the money from the sale, combined with small monthly

137

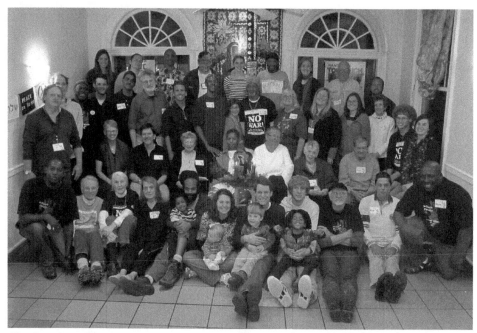

The Open Door Community was always at its liveliest when children were present. In this photo after Advent worship in 2011, Califf Johnson is in the front row with his younger son, Axe. His older son, Oxala, is in the lap of Eric Rucker (fourth from right). In the center front are Suzanne and Joseph Hobby Shippen and their sons, Benjamin and baby Michael. Both boys were baptized at the Open Door. Photo by Murphy Davis

Social Security payments and a little money from limited pension funds from our few early years of paid employment.

Our beloved Dayspring was a challenge to sell. We had transformed it from a family farm into a small retreat center that could sleep 30 people. After several months of hard effort, graciously overseen by Hannah, we finally had a buyer – if we agreed to finance the sale ourselves. The monthly payments we receive from that sale are a regular contribution we rely on to support the Open Door's ongoing ministry in Baltimore, for which we're grateful.

We parceled out our extensive theology and Black history library. We invited our many volunteers to take what they wanted of our African-American art and posters, drawings and paintings by death row prisoners, and our portrait gallery of community members and people on the streets – all large photographs lovingly made by Calvin and showcased with museum-quality framing. We had lived with and loved all of this, but we didn't have enough wall space in all our new homes combined for even a fraction of it.

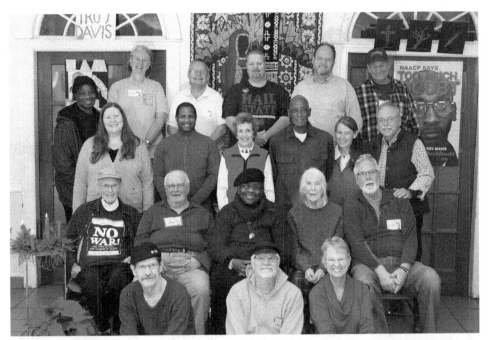

The community that worked to close the door and clear the house and Dayspring Farm gathered for the final Open Door photo in Atlanta. Back row: Sherry Morgan, Connie Bonner, Tim Mellen, David Payne, Ben Smith, Winston Robards. Row 3: Mary Catherine Johnson, Robert Lee, Anne Wheeler, James Walker, Julia Brook, Houston Wheeler. Row 2: Dick Rustay, Peter Vogelsang, Catherine Meeks, Gladys Rustay, Clive Bonner. Front row: David Christian, Ed Loring, Murphy Davis. Photo by Clive Bonner

The Special Collections division at Emory University received our archives. We handed over 35 years' worth of scrapbooks, letters, flyers, articles, and editions of *Hospitality*. With great dismay, we discovered that during the packing up of the house, tens of thousands of photographs documenting our history had been inadvertently thrown away. That's a loss that still continues to break my heart.

The task of packing up 910 Ponce de Leon and three buildings at Dayspring was exhausting both physically and emotionally. It seemed so difficult at times that I thought we wouldn't – *couldn't* – make it. But phenomenal help stepped forward and carried us through.

Beloved friends Connie and Clive Bonner came all the way from Scotland and spent three months helping us. Cordell Collier, who had lived in our yard and then in the community for a while – who always bought a get-well card and got everyone in the shower and soup-kitchen lines to sign it every time I went into the hospital – moved back in to help. Mary Jo Pfander, a dear friend in her late 70s, drove all the way from Ohio and showed up announcing, "I'm deaf as a doorknob, but I'm a very good organizer." We knew that to be

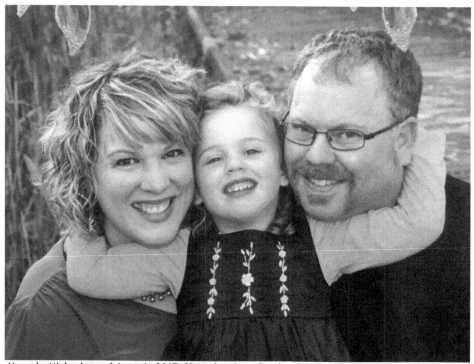

Hannah, Michaela, and Jason in 2017. Photo by Alison Reader, Framing Faces

true, and she graciously took on one task after another.

Lee and Rick Miller, rock-solid supporters of the Open Door through the years, gave us many hours of their time. Lee was renowned at their church, St. Anne's Episcopal, for dressing up like a turkey every year on a Sunday in early November. She would announce, "If you all bring frozen turkeys next Sunday, I won't do this again." In that way, she managed to get as many as 50 turkeys donated to serve 300 people at the Open Door on the day after Thanksgiving, when homeless people were still hungry and no other church was serving. Her effort prompted Ed to comment on there being "more turkeys than Christians" in a lot of churches around Thanksgiving.

My siblings Les, Mac, and Dot pitched in. So did Ben Smith, a one-time reporter who had covered our Imperial Hotel occupation, and Nibs Stroupe and Caroline Leach, Presbyterian pastors and generous friends. In the last days our good friends Carlton Mackey, of Emory University's Center for Ethics, and Kari Mackey, from the Carter Center, joined them. And David Payne and Robert Lee of our Open Door household worked tirelessly throughout.

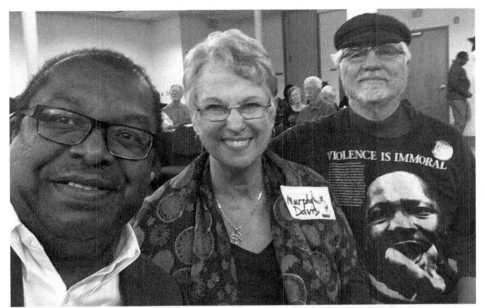

Ed and Murphy were honored by the Coalition for the Peoples Agenda with a celebratory lunch just before Christmas 2016, affording them an opportunity to say goodbye to many long-time colleagues in the Atlanta civil rights community, including dear friend Rev. Timothy McDonald (left). Selfie photo by Timothy McDonald

Tim Mellen, an old friend we had met through the Prison and Jail Project and Catholic Worker connections and hadn't seen in several years, came in December to spend two weeks with us. He had a gift for seeing what needed to be done and worked so hard that we asked if he would stay through Christmas. Once Christmas had come and gone, we asked if he would stay through the closing festivities. Long after we left, Tim was still there, taking care of the building until it was turned over to the new owners.

We definitely would not have made it through without the generosity of these special friends – and too many others to name. We had visits from friends near and far in the months before we closed. People came back to help, to touch base, to remember and share their stories. A few told us that they had cried when they got our letter about the Open Door closing. The sadness was almost overwhelming as we had our last soup kitchen, our last clinic, our last worship service. And then our final Christmas with all of our Open Door traditions.

The second weekend of January 2017, we hosted a celebration of all that had been, filled with music and storytelling. Friends came to Atlanta from all over the country, and our good friend Dietrich

Gerstner traveled all the way from Hamburg, Germany, where he and his wife Uta had established *Brot und Rosen* (Bread and Roses) Catholic Worker Community to harbor refugees. On Sunday evening we gathered downtown at Central Presbyterian Church for a poignant final communion service, followed by a simple feast.

The last thing we did was to march around the State Capitol Building, something we had done many times in three-and-a-half decades. We carried signs and banners from all our work through the years – protests against the death penalty and the vagrant-free zone, campaigns in support of public toilets and Grady Hospital. We sang and chanted "We're leaving, but the work is not done." We wanted to remind ourselves and our friends that, though things change, the work of clamoring for justice is never finished.

I so regretted that I was not feeling well during that weekend. I assumed that exhaustion had caught up with me again. The following week I discovered a suspicious bump on my scalp. *As if we need any more complications*, I thought. I called the Emory dermatology clinic. The first available appointment was February 18th, a month away and three days after our planned move to Baltimore.

Worried that the bump was something serious, I called Nicholas Beaulieu, "Dr. Nick," as we called him. He had worked in our soup kitchen when he was an Emory undergraduate and lived in our neighborhood. He had been extremely helpful when a mentally ill man who was high on something socked Ed in the eye. Nick had quickly sewed up the wound, saving us an entire day of waiting at Grady to get it taken care of.

He seemed always ready to help us. And that day he paved the way for me to see Amy Hatfield, his nurse practitioner, who treated the infection on my scalp with an antibiotic. But she knew there was more going on and encouraged me to see a dermatologist as soon as possible. So I called the Emory clinic every morning, hoping for a cancelled appointment that would open a space for me.

I guess they got tired of my daily call and, finally, on February 14th, I saw Dr. Feldman. When he pulled back my hair, he gasped, "That's not an infection, it's a tumor." It was an infection as well, but clearly the tumor was of greater concern to him. He told me I needed to get it removed right away. I said I was moving to Baltimore the next day. He went down the hall and got two surgeons. They gave me a shot and scooped out what they could, then wrapped my head in a big bandage. Dr. Feldman thought that the tumor was likely squamous cell cancer. But given my history, he was concerned that it might be lymphoma and told me to get medical attention as soon as I got to Baltimore.

Hannah had flown down to help with the final packing. In the end, with time and energy running out, we tossed a lot of stuff into boxes to sort out in Baltimore. These we crammed into two huge portable storage pods, along with our personal furniture and other possessions heading north. The next day all of us from the Open Door had dinner at Mary Mac's, one of Atlanta's best soul food restaurants, for our final time together. I swathed my large head bandage in a colorful scarf for the occasion and tried to trust that goodness and mercy would surely follow all of us to our new homes.

We had all realized that the 10-hour-plus van ride to Baltimore would be too much for me, so Ed dropped Hannah and me at the airport. Nibs Stroupe generously agreed to drive with Ed in the van. Robert Lee and David Payne had decided to join us in the new venture in Baltimore, and Robert drove our station wagon. David joined us a couple months later.

We rented a small house that Hannah and Jason had bought, close to them, with Ed and me living downstairs and David and Robert upstairs. David is an invaluable friend, working tirelessly in good spirits to keep our home and finances in order. Robert reconnected with family a few months after our arrival and moved to Florida. With Robert gone, we designated his room as a "Christ room" for hospitality and welcomed Simon, a gentle, generous Nigerian refugee who continues to make his home with us.

We were exhausted and in total chaos for a while, in a house full of boxes. The first week was agonizing as I waited for the results on the tumor. I didn't learn until Tuesday the 21st that it was in fact squamous cell and *not* lymphoma. Relieved by this news, I tackled my most pressing priority: to visit the Social Security office in Baltimore and transfer my Georgia Medicaid to Maryland. The man I spoke with there assured me that he could easily take care of the transfer, for which I was enormously grateful and once again relieved.

Because Hannah had worked in the Surgical ICU at Johns Hopkins Hospital for six years, she was able to pull a few strings to get the medical process started there for me. I had blood work and scans.

I quickly saw hematologist Nina Wagner-Johnson and dermatologist Robert Egbers. Concerned that the tumor was so large that it may have penetrated my skull, Dr. Egbers referred me to Carol Fackery, a head-and-neck cancer surgeon, and Sean Desai, a "plastic and rearrangement" surgeon. I'm glad I didn't realize at the time just how much "rearrangement" I was going to need. I knew that Johns Hopkins has some of the smartest doctors in the world, but I was not expecting the warm and compassionate response I received from all of these wonderful physicians.

The cancer had infiltrated the nerves in my scalp. I needed an incredibly complex "flap surgery." I had to have it as soon as possible – and especially before mid-April, because Dr. Desai was getting married and leaving on his honeymoon then – and the surgery was so complicated that very few doctors in the world could do it.

The anguish of having to undergo a difficult major surgery in the midst of closing the Open Door and moving 700 miles away was aggravated by my health insurance situation. In early March I got a call from a woman – let's call her Celia – in the Johns Hopkins financial office. Celia informed me that I had no health insurance on record.

I told her that I had taken care of it at the Social Security office, and she replied, "Well, it's not showing up on the computer." She informed me that the cost would be $1,360 per day in the hospital – not including any medications or the surgery itself. "I don't know if you can have your surgery," she declared.

But I knew I needed it ASAP. I spoke about my dilemma with Dr. Barbara Cook, a member of Brown Memorial Park Avenue Presbyterian Church, where Ed and I had been attending with Hannah and Michaela. A retired physician and administrator, Barbara had gone back to work with the foundation that oversees issues with patients who are uninsured or underinsured. She is a wizard with such thorny problems. She told me not to cancel any appointments and put a couple of her co-workers on the case.

Celia called at 8 o'clock each morning to see if there was any progress. "I'm gonna have to qualify you as self-pay," she finally told me one day with exasperation. "Before you have the surgery, you're gonna have to come down here to the financial office with three hundred and nine thousand, one hundred and fifty-one dollars and seventy-three cents."

I said to her, "Celia, do you think I should laugh or cry?" I wish now that I had gone down there and handed her the 73 cents and said, "We'll be back with the rest after we rob a bank."

I made a visit to the Baltimore Social Services office, a huge room crowded with about a hundred people in all stages of repair and disrepair. I took a number and a seat. Eventually I was called to the desk of an older African-American woman, who had been there a few decades, knew the system, and clearly did *not* suffer fools. When I explained the problem, she considered it an emergency and dove right into getting to the bottom of it, immediately firing off an email to the man I had spoken with at the Social Security office. He had never sent over my paperwork.

"You're gonna be okay," she assured me, and the knots in my stomach began to untangle. She got me on Maryland Medicaid just in the nick of time.

The surgeons worked in two stages. On March 20th they cut out the tumor. They covered the resulting hole in my head with a strip of Integra, a wound dressing made of silicone and bovine tendon collagen, designed to mimic human skin. Ed lovingly referred to the thick protrusion on my scalp as my "cowhide pillbox hat."

On April 4th, the surgeons took a deep slice of my forearm and grafted it onto my head. Making a trench down the side of my face in front my right ear, a second set of surgeons connected the arm graft's arteries and veins into my body's vascular system under my jaw, to ensure that plenty of blood flowed to the head wound. The arteries presented no problems, but the doctors had to work for hours to connect the small veins, which had been weakened by chemotherapy and showed signs of deterioration. Just as they got one vein connected, another would "blow" and they had to start all over again. Once everything was in place, they cut a four-by-six-inch patch of skin from my left thigh and grafted it onto the hole in my forearm.

After the surgery Dr. Desai walked into the waiting room and plopped into a chair across from Ed, Hannah, and Lee Miller, who had come from Atlanta to help out. He had been on his feet for eight hours. They reported that he was the most exhausted doctor they had ever seen. Knowing that he could have given up at several points but didn't, the good doctor and I both teared up during my emotional thank-you to him later.

I came out of the surgery with three large, gaping wounds – on my head, on my forearm, and on my thigh. I looked and felt like a

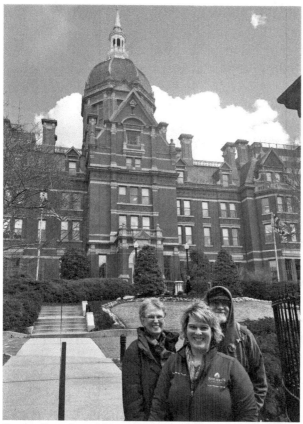

Murphy, Hannah, and Ed stop in front of the oldest building of Johns Hopkins Hospital in February 2017 as they work to arrange Murphy's urgently needed flap surgery. Photo by unknown person passing by

piece of chopped meat. I spent the first 24 hours in the same surgical ICU where Hannah had worked, and then spent a week on a ward in the Weinberg Cancer Center. Dr. Desai visited every day, carefully cleaning the blood crusting around my wounds. "Can I believe my eyes?" a nurse asked in wonderment after he left. She had never before seen a surgeon take the time to clean a wound.

All kinds of things could have gone wrong, and a resident who was concerned about the look of my wounds on Saturday night, four days after my surgery, took pictures and sent them to Dr. Desai. His wedding was a week away, and his relatives from India had arrived for the celebration, but he drove 45 minutes from his home to check on me. When I apologized for the interruption, he said with a shy grin, "It's okay. We were doing gift bags. I think they'll be just fine without me." After being satisfied that everything was all right, he walked out the door anticipating his Christian-Hindu wedding – complete with his riding into the ceremony on a horse – and I thought about how blessed the young woman is who gets to spend her life with this brilliant and kind doctor.

Once I was home, Hannah came every single day to care for my gruesome wounds, as she had after my first surgery when she was 15. It was a repeated act of extraordinary love, especially given that she was by then a spouse, a full-time nursing instructor, a Ph.D. student, and the mother of a toddler. Her vigilant care to ward off infection was the only reason I didn't have to be re-hospitalized after the surgery. At the expense of her own family, Hannah kept me alive.

Michaela was the sunshine that kept us all going. Every day she showed up with a parade of dolls and stuffed animals – all with head wounds. She wrapped their heads in bandages and rushed them to the "hostible" for surgery. She confessed to her mother later, "I know it's *hospital*, but I say *hostible* because you all think it's so funny."

Hannah gave Michaela the very important role of being her assistant, and

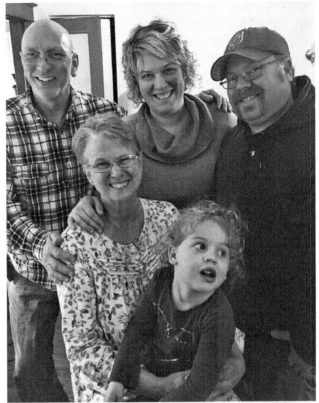

Andrew Legare (top left), a dear friend ever since he was sentenced to death in Georgia in 1977, is one of the rare persons released from death row. After 27 years in prison, he rejoined his beloved wife, Mary Palmer Legare, and lives not too far from Murphy and Ed, allowing frequent visits. In March 2017 he gathered with Hannah, Jason, and Michaela around Murphy as Hannah got ready to shave her mother's head in preparation for surgery the next morning to remove the tumor from her scalp. Photo by Ed Loring

Michaela carefully cut gauze and lined up supplies. I was moved by Hannah's sensitivity to Michaela's need to be involved, so as not to be terrified by my wounds and grisly appearance.

For me, the role of "Mamotes," my chosen grandmother name, was an unending source of joy in that most difficult time. I recovered the name from my childhood. When I was young, I was known as Martha Murphy. I was named after my Dad's sister, who was named Martha after their grandmother (though she went by Mattie). My second name came from my Uncle Murph, my mother's brother, who was named after their father (both of whom baptized me when I was an infant). As a small child,

147

Murph's son, my cousin Robin Williams, had trouble pronouncing "Martha Murphy" (can you blame him?). It came out as "Mamotes," which became a term of endearment used for a while for me by my mother and Robin's. It felt right to revive it all these years later as my grandmother name.

I needed radiation on my scalp after the surgery to ensure that all the cancer disappeared, but it was a tough call for the doctors. Doing it too early would destroy the skin graft; too late, and the cancer was likely to return. Again and again they delayed, giving my wounded head a little more time to heal. Finally, in the middle of June, I had four weeks of it, feeling lousy as I always did on radiation. But, remarkably, I began to feel better in August and the multiple wounds in my body slowly healed.

Other crises visited us in Baltimore over time, seemingly endless. I got a whopper of a kidney infection that took me to the Johns Hopkins Emergency Room. I hovered on the edge of sepsis and once again came close to dying, but was rescued by IV antibiotics. Ed had a serious bike accident while on his way to officiate with me at the wedding of our good friend Vicky and her undocumented sweetheart. He broke his wrist in five places and had to have metal plates surgically implanted. The pain was excruciating and the swelling in his hand so severe that Jason had to saw off his wedding ring.

A couple days later I experienced – yet again – crippling abdominal pain, was rushed to the ER, and was told I had gallstones. This seemed impossible. Though I remembered very little about it afterward, I was quite sure that

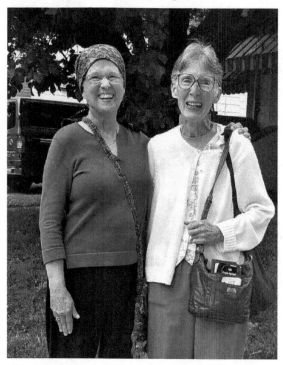

Several close friends came to help Ed and Murphy during her recuperation from the flap surgery. Mary Sinclair came twice, and her quiet presence was a balm for weary spirits. Photo by Ed Loring

I had had my gall bladder surgically removed a few years earlier. But apparently some of it got missed the first time, and so I got to have it taken out a second time – bringing the tally of scars across my torso to an even two vertical and two horizontal.

In February 2018, 910 Ponce de Leon was demolished. It was, as former Open Door resident volunteer Nathan Dorris described it, "torn down, reduced to a pile of rubble, swept up and taken God knows where." Nathan wrote his reflections on the demolition in the March 2018 issue of *Hospitality*. He acknowledged that many well-intended friends, anxious to offer comfort, spoke about the Open Door living

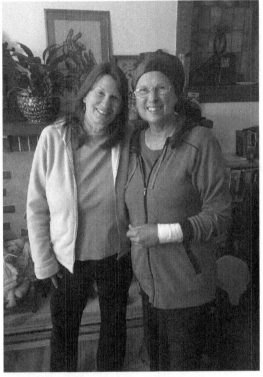

Joyce Hollyday always seems to find a way to come and help, and her visits filled with gifts of cooking, cleaning, transportation, stimulating conversation, and lots of laughs, have kept Murphy and Ed going. Photo by Ed Loring

on in the hearts and minds of those of us who had shared life there and the thousands of people we had served. But he encouraged sitting for a while with "the pain of desecration":

That land – those bricks, those trees, even that concrete – has for the last thirty-odd years been soaking every aspect of the life of that community into itself. There are actual drops of blood, sweat and tears in more than one place on those premises. It is holy ground, a bush alight... Water from showers offered and given freely to those otherwise denied a place to wash themselves ran across smooth tile, seeped into porous stone; coffee made with love (and mountains of sugar) poured out as libation upon earth and woodchips in the front yard. The thousands upon thousands of voices sharing their thoughts or feelings, singing loudly, poorly, earnestly, etching themselves into the leaves of the trees or the notches in the benches.

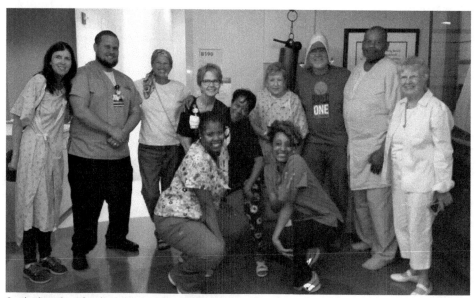

On the last day of radiation treatments, each patient is invited to "ring the bell" on the way home. Robin (center) and Murphy finished on the same day in July 2017, and everyone - patients, partners, and staff - gathered for the ringing of the bell and big hugs and thanksgiving. One patient was from Chicago, and another came from Argentina with her family. Johns Hopkins waiting rooms are always an international experience waiting to become a community of support and care. Photo by radiation oncology staff person

I still grieve that the Open Door's former home no longer exists in Atlanta. I miss eating supper with a diverse family, our worship, the Eucharist we shared, our music. Our little house band was a joy. I think often of Dick, a classically trained clarinetist who could bend a note 'til it was blue all over; Calvin on his banjo, making every musical moment a sing-along; and Mike, who often cut loose on the piano with his considerable talent and characteristic sense of fun. Nelia and I collaborated in creating our Sunday night community liturgy. Gladys made sure all the bulletins and songbooks were in place, and of course Ed was always ready to preach, shout, and greet our guests. We haven't yet found a faith community with the depth of experience we were able to create together in Atlanta. It's what all six of us miss about our life together more than anything else.

I continue to be plagued with numerous health complications related to all the chemo and radiation to which my body has been subjected, the ravages of the fungal pneumonia, and my compromised immune system. Most recently, I face diminished energy as a result of a chronic lung infection and congestive heart failure. I still have IV infusions to boost my immune system every few weeks, and I take a pharmacy's worth of medications. I'm grateful for every drug and dose that helps to keep me alive.

Medical science is always revealing new insights about how our bodies work and interact with medications. Dr. Manisha Loss, another of my new doctors and a brilliant research dermatologist, discovered in collaboration with other researchers a relationship between Voraconazole and the rapid growth of squamous cell cancers. Voraconazole, in its former form of Posaconazole, saved my life when I had fungal pneumonia in 2004, and it continued for almost a decade and a half to keep the disease in check. But it also began causing out-of-control growth of squamous cell tumors around the edges of my face. My doctors took me off the drug.

In November 2018 I had another large tumor on my hairline surgically removed. Time for another "rearrangement" with Dr. Desai. He made incisions that enabled him to stretch my radiated skin, leaving a hole that was much smaller but still left a piece of my skull exposed. When the wound still wasn't fully healed weeks later, he said that a second surgery might be necessary. I dreaded hearing those words and begged for more time to try to find another solution. I met with dozens of nurses and, finally, with the help of one of Hannah's friends, found the Center for Wound Healing at Howard County General Hospital, affiliated with Johns Hopkins.

Hope seemed to follow Dr. Hadley Katherine Wesson around. I felt it when she came into the room on our first visit. She introduced a new product called A-Cell that she wanted to use on my forehead wound. It was a powder made from the lining of a pig's bladder. *Well, why not?* I already had cow tendons on my head, why not a pig's bladder too?

And so I saw Dr. Wesson for a treatment every Wednesday afternoon from February to August in 2019. It was a 70-mile round-trip drive for Ed and me each week, but the healing gradually was accomplished. We got to know Dr. Wesson and the nurses in the clinic very well, and we knew we would miss them when the treatments were over. At my last appointment, we had a little "Pig Party," complete with cupcakes bearing the likeness of pig faces in the frosting and purple socks emblazoned with flying pink pigs for everybody.

Since January 1, 2018, Ed and David have faithfully served an early breakfast twice a week outside a subway station in poverty-ravaged West Baltimore, the neighborhood where Freddie Gray was killed by Baltimore police. On that first day, David and Ed handed a granola bar and a cup of coffee to six guests. Now a couple hundred show up to be served at The Welcome Table, in the space that Ed has named the Upton Underground Railway Station, in honor of Harriet Tubman, a Marylander who is well known and highly honored in our city.

David and Ed are joined by Deacon Ty Cole and Sister Erica Prettyman of Newborn Community Faith Church. They both bring a loyal and loving spirit to the breakfast, and Ed and David often say how much they treasure them. Erica is "The Soup Lady," famous on the streets for her hot, thick chicken noodle soup, which she generously ladles out to people who wait in long lines to receive it. Without fail, guests sing its praises, and they generally appreciate the granola bar, banana, and coffee offered as well – though, as in Atlanta, some find that three cups of sugar per hundred cups of coffee just isn't enough.

Erica, Ty, David, Ed, and Beth Dellow, an active Episcopalian laywoman who recently joined them, serve breakfast in the blistering heat and thick humidity of Baltimore's summers. And they serve it in the blasting frigidness of its winters. One day in January 2019, the wind chill factor was three degrees below zero. It was so cold that when Ed tried to start the van after the breakfast, his hands were too numb to turn the key.

Gusts were blowing at 20 miles an hour that morning. The tops of the soup pots "clashed like cymbals," according to Ed, and then went rolling down the street, as napkins, cups, and spoons shot into the air and scattered everywhere. Everyone pitched in to gather it all back up. And then Erica, Ty, David, and Ed carried on, serving people who had no warm place to go for escape from the cold, no shelter from the stormy blasts.

Though things change, the work of clamoring for justice is never finished.

12

'Remember that You Are Dust...'

Every Ash Wednesday at the Open Door Community in Atlanta, we gathered in the early morning around a big soup pot filled with twigs and crumpled newspaper in our backyard. This was as close as we could get to having a fire pit in downtown Atlanta. We read together the words of the 51st Psalm, in Nan Merrill's wonderful adaptation, *Psalms for Praying*:

> *Have mercy on me, O Gracious One,*
> > *according to your steadfast love...*
> *Forgive all that binds me in fear,*
> > *that I might radiate love...*
> *Look not on my past mistakes*
> > *but on the aspirations of my heart.*
> *Create in me a clean heart...*
> *Restore in me the joy of your saving grace,*
> > *and encourage me with a new spirit.*

After the reading, we meditated silently on our own brokenness and the places in our lives where we needed to receive God's mercy and transformation. We wrote these down on small pieces of paper and laid our confessions in the soup pot. Dick Rustay then struck a match and lit the pile of paper. When the blaze died to cool embers, he carefully stirred the ashes, reached in, turned, and marked the forehead of the person standing beside him. Then one by one around the circle, we bestowed the sign of the cross with the ashes and the words "Remember that you are dust, and to dust you will return."

Dust. Our bodies are made of the "stuff" of the earth – the raw matter also known as *humus*. It is the root of our word *humility*.

Our bodies connect us to the earth of which we are a part. To be humble is to stand with bare feet on the earth and feel its rhythms. To remember that we are connected to the entire web of life. We are not separate or "above" the rest of creation; we are a part of it all.

In modern technological culture, we suffer the illusion that we can live in our minds, cut off from the earth. But when our bodies become ill, we are forced to remember from whence we came. They carry memories that our minds have not received.

In the labor of illness, these "body memories" can come to us: the tears and blood of the ancestors that have soaked the earth beneath us; the poisoning and rape of the land; the slaughter of the creatures. Though our bodies also carry the memory of those who have loved the earth and tended it well, in our era of technological frenzy the earth cries out to us, and its pleas most often fall on ears rendered unable to hear by the frantic life of market capitalism and its voracious appetites. The illnesses that afflict our bodies are not apart from the devastation and weeping of the earth itself.

Someone once said that illness is "God's reset button." Illness can be an occasion for us to wake up. And if the diagnosis takes us to the very brink of death, the awakening is monumental indeed. A critical illness will change us in some way, but it does not necessarily change us one way or another. It is possible that a person can be changed into a self-pitying hypochondriac, with illness as their vocation, the center of life and self-concern. But critical illness can also be an opportunity to grow in wisdom and love. Illness is a crucible, a refining fire. It has a way, if we listen carefully, of burning away all that does not matter – all the dross, fear, materialism, and resentment, all the petty concerns and irritations – so that all that remains is gratitude.

Despite all the dire predictions, I am alive. I am grateful. But I am grateful not only for the extension of my life; I am most deeply grateful for a new understanding of the power of life that comes when days are numbered. One gift of illness – when life is measured out in pills and doses and regimens – is that it forces us to live in the present, moment by moment. Part of the miracle of life unfolding day by day is learning what a gift is *each* day. How deep and rich and sacramental is that gift!

I get weary, but I've never said I've had enough. I love life, and I sometimes feel that I could *never* get enough. Though my energy is very limited, I keep waking up every day and doing what I can: editing and writing for *Hospitality*, corresponding with friends in prison, attending events of the Poor People's Campaign in Baltimore and protest vigils in Washington, D.C., with Ed as I'm able. And I *always* find the energy for Michaela, who visits often and stays overnight with us at least one night every week. She keeps our hearts entertained and our spirits lifted by telling us imaginative stories, regaling us with all that she's learning in her Montessori school, and playing songs on the piano. "Yankee Doodle Dandy," which she played in a recent recital, is a current favorite.

I wear four long scars – two that run the length of my torso and two that cross my abdomen left to right – plus countless smaller ones, straight, curved, and round. They remind me day in and day out that four times my body had to be laid open for my life to be spared, and multiple other times cancer and infection were removed in smaller doses. On nine separate occasions, the skilled hands and well-trained eyes of dedicated surgeons took from me what was unneeded and hurtful and left the vital parts restored to health. All of this drastic cutting and sewing and stapling has saved my life. The scars are constant reminders that it is always time for gratitude.

I've beaten the odds again and again. But I know that this will not always be so. I feel deep in my lungs and down to my bones how compromised my body is by 25 years of assaults upon it. I know that repeated chemotherapy and radiation have affected my energy and my mental focus. I have not died on anybody's medical timetable but, like everyone, I *will* die.

During the hours that Ed and I walked with our friend Jack Alderman through death watch in September 2008, he shared a story with us. After he had received word of his execution date, a prison guard stopped him in the hallway and asked, "Well, Jack, are you ready?" Jack's response was quick and clear: "Hell, no, I'm not ready...But I'm *prepared*."

I'm with Jack. I might not ever be ready. But I hope I'm prepared.

When I ponder my dying, I think most of Michaela. Of course I would love to be around to watch this precious child I'm so close to grow up, as I had prayed so fervently to watch her mother mature into adulthood. But I also recognize that Michaela, now 6 years old, is at a tender age. We have a special and beautiful relationship, and I would like her to remember me this way – not as someone she has to watch decline mentally and physically. I want her to remember me always as *this* version of Mamotes. I don't want to turn into somebody else.

And so I know that I probably will not subject my body and my soul and my family to any more prolonged treatment or any extraordinary life-saving measures. I have a daughter who is a skilled and compassionate expert in palliative and end-of-life care. In contrast to the many people I've watched die who had been judged unworthy to live, I know that I will be extravagantly loved into death, by a remarkable partner and a myriad of family members and friends.

I also know that, as surely as I am stalked by death, I am also stalked by goodness and mercy. They are following, pursuing, chasing, running after me. And they will never stop. Even when I leave this world. I don't know how long I have left to stay here, but I do know I'm under a deadline – and I've always needed a deadline to get me moving! So I'm packing up, preparing, getting ready.

It is one of the great paradoxes of the life of faith that when we are truly prepared to die, we can authentically choose life. Part of the task of maturity is learning to live as one prepared to die. When we cling to life, anxious to hold on and pretending that we will cheat the inevitable end, then in fact we choose death. "Teach us to number our days," sings the Psalmist, "that we may gain a heart of wisdom" (Ps. 90:12). Otherwise translated: "Teach us how short life is that we may have a wise heart." Until we can face death, we do not begin to live fully and deeply.

Dr. Martin Luther King Jr. was a great teacher about facing death. His life was at tremendous risk from the moment he stepped up to the pulpit to assume leadership in the Montgomery Bus Boycott. He and his beloved young family endured hateful late-night phone calls, terrifying threats, the bombing of their home. Dr. King and everyone around him knew that it was just a matter of time before an assassin would hit the target. In response to this truth, he reflected: "Our lives begin to end the day we become silent about things that matter."

While our situations differ in the particulars, we each face the same choice: Will I, or will I not, live every day as one prepared to die?

Memento mori is a Latin phrase translated "Remember you will die." While it may sound morbid to our 21st-century ears, it is ancient wisdom about the path to becoming fully human. Those who have meditated on this truth through the ages have done so not to promote fear, but to inspire and make clear the transient nature of this earthly life and its possessions and pursuits. Though our capacity for denial is remarkable, death is the one absolute certainty in life. Nobody ever gets out of this world alive, and the sooner we can face and make peace with our own deaths, the sooner we can begin to live at the deepest level.

At one of my lowest points, I wrote in my journal: "I feel in my battered flesh the measure of my days. I see in my jagged scars the journey of fighting for the goodness of life." What I know in the depth of my being is that this journey is one that requires community. The love of family and friends fills my life and crowds out the fear. It is like a warm blanket wrapped forever around me.

Hannah has reminded me on occasion that the abundance of the love doesn't mean that *she* is not afraid. She and Ed struggle in a way that I do not with the fear of my death and dying. They are the ones who will be left behind. So there is a very real sense that my task is an easier one. But I think it's safe to say that none of us would have made it, and we all would have been overwhelmed by the fear, except for the love: the great, faithful, ever-present love of those who stand by us and with us and mediate the loving grace of God.

Maintaining hope alone while facing mortality and embracing fragility is very difficult, if not impossible. When my hope flags, I need you to be hopeful. And you need me, in your hardest times, to lend you my hope. I learned from an elder many years ago that when we work to keep hope alive in someone else, we find that it keeps it alive in ourselves.

All through my illness, time and time again, my community prayed its heart out for me – for my healing, that I might not be overwhelmed by my physical suffering, that my doctors would have the best wisdom to know how to help me through. I have been saved, over and over, by the prayers of the poor. Their hope surrounded and buoyed me. And it was contagious.

"Hope is the simplest trust that God has not forgotten the recipe for manna." I love these words from W. Paul Jones in his book on Christian spirituality, *Trumpet at Full Moon*. Manna was the promise and fulfillment of God's provision to our ancestors in the wilderness. It was digestible hope. For 40 years it appeared every morning, sustenance from a God who could be trusted to show up.

Manna was also a sign of God's justice, a promise not to individuals but to a *community*. As long as every person and family took only what they needed, the abundance was shared and all was well. But when some members of the community took more than their fair share – when they decided to accumulate and hoard – the manna "bred worms and became foul" (Ex. 16:20). Manna was a lesson in how to meet the needs of all and live for the common good.

But the lesson was quickly forgotten. Once they reached the Promised Land, our ancestors in the faith let human nature take over. Before long, great inequalities in wealth took hold. The hoarders prospered on their vast estates while the poor suffered in their tiny hovels. Debt slavery, labor exploitation, hunger, illness, and imprisonment became widespread: the price a society pays when life becomes defined by consuming and accumulating.

Years ago, just after a rash of teenage suicides in the wealthy East Cobb County area of suburban Atlanta, I was invited to address the students of the First Year Seminar at Mercer University. After speaking of the suffering of the homeless poor and the thousands of men, women, and children caged in Georgia's prisons, I asked the students: "Is there not some connection between the children in downtown Atlanta who are desperately poor, hungry, and homeless, and the children of affluence in East Cobb County who are taking their own lives?"

After my talk, many of the students stayed to ask questions and share their thoughts. One young man waited patiently and then said quietly, "I know why those kids in East Cobb are killing themselves." I asked him to say more. With a certainty that made clear he knew something about what he was talking about, he said, "They don't have any idea that they can be anything more than an appetite."

When we *become* our appetites, we fit quite nicely into a society that, as Oscar Wilde put it, "knows the price of everything and the value of nothing." We are infected with the hubris that makes us the center of our own existence. We live to consume, and eventually we consume each other and our very selves.

Consumption as a way of life is perhaps nowhere more dangerous than in our healthcare system – and it is most obvious in the care we dole out to the poorest of the poor. As Ed and I have made a new home in Baltimore, we've stayed connected to friends in Atlanta and paid special attention to developments at Grady Memorial Hospital, for which I remain grateful as each new year of life rolls around and I am still here.

We still consider the Grady Campaign one of our rare successes in a lifetime of struggles for justice. But, despite our effort and its good outcome, Grady continues to be an ominous symbol of the state of health care in this country. Just months after our campaign, the staff of pharmacists was reduced to less than a skeleton, and the main pharmacy, which normally served up to 1,000 patients per day, was giving out tickets to the first 200 to 400 in line. The rest were turned away by security guards. For many patients, such delays meant death or debilitating crisis that ultimately ended up costing the hospital much more in emergency care than timely treatment would have.

In spite of having the funds to run the hospital and provide for all its patients, Grady's administration allowed the situation to get worse and worse. Subsequent administrations in the past two decades did little better. One CEO left the position announcing – falsely – that he had brought Grady to solvency and that "Atlanta should shine my shoes." *Wow. How insensitive can a wealthy white man be?* Friends in Atlanta report improvements in services under the current hospital administration, but it is no secret that there has been a political agenda in some quarters for several years to dismantle Grady – either to run off the poor patients and privatize the hospital, or just to let the system collapse on itself.

The crisis at Grady is part of a larger national agenda to consolidate power and privilege for the wealthy and take from the poor what little they have had in the way of goods, services, and dignity. "Safety net" hospitals have been increasingly under assault from the political Right. Beginning with the era of Ronald Reagan's presidency, it has become more and more permissible to publicly mock and even hate the "undeserving poor" – especially the Black and Brown poor.

Reagan's eight years in the White House established a solid movement for those working to reverse the progress brought about by the civil rights struggle, and even the earlier social guarantees of Franklin Roosevelt's New Deal. This movement has been consolidated in a highly effective, systematic backlash. It has co-opted practically all of our national leadership – Republican *and* Democratic.

Since the early 1980s, a steady and persistent legislative and judicial agenda has given virtually every advantage to wealthy individuals, corporations, and institutions, while handing crushing disadvantages to working-class and poor people. Public institutions and services have been opened up to the forces of privatization for the purpose of increasing profits for the already-wealthy, creating a destabilized environment for workers. At the same time, at national, state, and local levels, virtually every program that in any way helps the poor has been cut back or gutted entirely.

During the presidency of Bill Clinton, two pieces of federal legislation, the Welfare Reform Act of 1996 and the Balanced Budget Act of 1997, cut loose many of our most vulnerable citizens, compromising or abolishing the programs that ensured their survival. The bills were devastating to public hospitals and their patients. As people were moved "from welfare to work," they more often than not ended up in low-wage, dead-end jobs that almost never provided health insurance. More recently, many states – under Republican leadership determined to undermine the Affordable Care Act ("Obamacare") – have refused its provision for Medicaid expansion, depriving millions of poor people of health coverage and dooming many to debility or death.

In these decades the United States has undergone massive and sweeping change that has increasingly consolidated resources and put them in fewer and fewer hands. People in the wealthiest 1 percent have amassed personal fortunes in the millions and billions – more than the annual budgets of some of the world's nations. While they accumulate more money and possessions than anybody could ever need in a lifetime, the middle class is more vulnerable, the working class is close to falling over the edge, and the poor have sunk more and more deeply into the misery of substandard housing, homelessness, predatory lending, prison, and limited access to good schools, proper nutrition, and life-sustaining health care.

Simply put, the emergency we're in has been created by specific policy decisions at every level of government over a period of many years. Some folks knew doggone well what they were doing, a few people protested in vain, and the rest seemed to be watching TV or shopping at the mall. But as all of the cuts continue to trickle down to the local level, they are deadly for the poor, the sick, and the vulnerable.

Thanks to Obamacare, the number of people without health insurance in the U.S. decreased from more than 44 million in 2013 to just below 27 million in 2016. But due to ongoing efforts to undermine the Affordable Care Act and put restrictions on Medicaid, the number has started to climb again – by approximately 125,000 people each month.

The price for Posaconazole, the anti-fungal drug that saved my life, and its successor Voraconazole, which sustained me for 15 years, hovered around $3,000 per month. This drug – and the tests, hospitalizations, surgeries, follow-up appointments, infusions, and other medications that have kept me alive – have been largely covered by Medicaid Disability and more recently, Medicare. But what about those who need such care and have been rejected by the Disability system?

As Medicaid has been threatened and cut over the years, my participation in advocacy has continued to be a very personal agenda. The personal is indeed political; the political is indeed personal. Perhaps it is not so for people who can pay their way through any crisis, but for those who are poor – or who choose to be in solidarity with the poor – it must be.

Solidarity means doing the hard work of learning about our power, our privilege, and our assumptions. It involves what Ivan Illich called "de-schooling." Those of us who were born and bred of white supremacy were intentionally taught a worldview that was not – and is not – true. As painful as it is, we have to learn how much of what we accept as truth is not just "not quite right" but is built on intentional lies.

We can start by recognizing the real roots of our national story: the widespread slaughter of Native peoples from coast to coast over land and resources, and the enslavement of millions of Africans and their descendants as a source of free labor, enforced through exploitation, family separation, torture, and rape on a massive scale. We are inheritors of this legacy – which continued through forced removal to reservations, Jim Crow segregation and lynchings, debt slavery, denial of education and loans – and persists today in multiple forms of racism and discrimination. It shows up, among many other places, in how we treat the poor in our medical system.

According to several recent studies, we in the United States spend more than $10,000 per person per year on health care. This is twice what other industrialized countries spend on average – and they have healthcare systems that provide access to care for *all* their citizens. Despite our enormous expenditure, we cannot claim to have the best health care – or the best health – in the world. In countries with universal national healthcare, infant mortality rates are lower and life expectancy is longer. This is related to both guaranteed access and a lack of anxiety and stress about getting needed treatment and medications.

For all our expenditures of government and private money, we are getting less for more. So why don't we, like Canada and Great Britain and all the other industrialized nations on the globe, move immediately to a national health plan? The answer seems to have something to do with the fact that the lion's share of our healthcare dollars are pouring into enormous corporate profits. This includes huge government subsidies for a healthcare system that moves public money into private coffers rather than toward the common good. We are paying through the nose to maintain the obscene wealth of the elite rather than the general health of the people.

Dr. David Hilfiker, a compassionate and inspiring physician who has spent most of his career working with homeless people and those dying from AIDS in Washington, D.C., used a disturbing term in his memoir *Not All of Us Are Saints*. Having observed the medical crisis in India that prompted the work of Mother Teresa, Hilfiker believes that we are headed toward the same disaster in this country: just let the sick poor wander our streets until they die their miserable deaths. He calls this "The Calcutta Solution."

Author Ayn Rand calls such ones in need "second handers." Her Republican disciples want to get rid of anything that might be helpful to those deemed "unworthy parasites." Many in our sick political arena can explain to you just why poverty or sickness is "their fault," because of "their bad choices." The climate continues to get meaner in the war on the poor.

The problem with our medical system is that the political mood of our country is raging toward narcissistic consumerism. It is assumed that there is a market answer to every question or dilemma, including health care. All services and institutions are becoming fair game for the market, and all space is becoming commercial space.

The values and language of the market have come to so dominate our common life that ethical discussion, and religious or moral discourse, have begun to seem at least quaint, if not completely irrelevant. The "bottom line" is everything. Those who matter are consumers. And poor people (by definition, without capital) are not consumers, so they literally don't count. In fact, they don't even exist, except as commodities in the prison-industrial complex. The Calcutta Solution indeed.

When I began writing this memoir more than two decades ago, I could not have imagined that in the week that I would finish it, India would declare a total lockdown of its country in response to the coronavirus pandemic – forcing tens of millions of city laborers out of work and launching a mass migration of people vulnerable to disease and starvation, desperate to get to their home villages and families. As I write these closing thoughts during the last week of March 2020, the U.S. is also hurtling toward total lockdown, ten million U.S. workers have filed for unemployment benefits as their jobs have disappeared, COVID-19 cases worldwide have surpassed a million, and 50,000 people have died from the disease. According to the experts at Johns Hopkins and elsewhere, this is just the beginning. The staggering reality is likely to be far worse by the time this book is printed. And, given the scientific evidence linking pandemics to climate change, we are likely to face this again and again.

I am sequestered at home, hyper-vigilant once more, unable for the time being to visit with Hannah and Michaela except by phone with facetime. I'm concerned about Jason and all the other emergency and medical workers on the front lines. I think of all the people crowded into prisons and those who don't have homes in which to shelter, or the means to stay fed and safe during this global crisis. And I'm deeply troubled – though not surprised – that the pandemic is disproportionately affecting people in poverty and communities of color.

In a Winship Cancer Center waiting room in 2009, Ed got into a conversation with a man from South Georgia while his wife and I were being prepped for chemotherapy infusions. Ed asked him what kind of work he did, and he began grumping about how hard it was to be a banker and developer during a recession. He then asked Ed what he did.

"I work with homeless people," Ed answered.

Immediately the banker said, "Oh, they're worthless."

"They are not!" shouted Ed, drawing some attention to the two of them.

Embarrassed, the man stammered, "I don't mean they're worthless people. I just mean they're worthless to the economy and the workforce."

The market-driven, for-profit system is intended to build the privilege of a few and increase a sense of powerlessness among the rest of us. The body politic appears to be in a stranglehold grip of paralysis and futility. The electoral process is so controlled by the same corporate interests that are reaping the benefits of this system that movement seems almost impossible.

But we do not have to accept the sense of powerlessness that we are intended to feel. The consolidation of power and resources demands privacy, secrecy, and the expectation that everybody will stay focused on their individual lives and wellbeing. As we learned during the Grady Campaign, the back-room deals can be publicly challenged, and the process of decision-making around the use of public resources can be forced into the open for public debate and accountability.

Matthew 25, so foundational and challenging to the life of the Open Door Community, forces us all to ask: Did we feed, serve, welcome, visit? Did we follow Jesus to the cells and soup lines, to the margins and borders, to the desolate places where he told us we could find him and his beloved sisters and brothers? He invites each of us to a life of compassion. *Compassion* means "to suffer with." It involves more than "doing good" for others. It calls for solidarity through shared suffering: because you are suffering, I am suffering.

Jesus gave us a definition of solidarity when he said, "No one has greater love than this, to lay down one's life for one's friends" (Jn. 15:13). We tend to spiritualize and individualize this call of Jesus into heroic and high drama of the sort that, frankly, most of us will never face. Giving our lives for our friends is instead the much more daily and mundane task of placing who we are and what we have – our resources, our time, our attention – at the service of the disinherited and those with their backs against the wall. Solidarity means stretching our hearts. It means giving things up – not once, or twice, but continually. It means forgoing privileges and conveniences that make things easier for us while leaving others to fend for themselves.

The solidarity that lives in us and binds us as people of faith means that the liberation of the poor is not simply a political agenda or an ideological program that we can pick up or lay aside at will. Solidarity means that we recognize the liberation of the poor as our life's agenda, because liberation clamors out from human history to the ears of God. This liberation is coming. It is promised. As Dr. King said, "The arc of the universe is long, but it bends toward justice."

The real question for each of us is: Which side am I on? We know the deepest joy when we struggle on behalf of others. It is not a question of what or how much we do to assist the poor, but whether or not we have given our lives over to a commitment to the poor as our family. The solidarity I experienced in my illness was not because of what I was doing – because I was not doing anything, for all appearances. Rather, the poor were taking care of me, welcoming me into *their* space. I am most alive when I fight for the lives of the poor as if it were my own life – because it *is* my own life.

Solidarity is the relationship for which we are created. The path of solidarity ultimately leads to the Oneness of God and creation, the mystical Body of Christ that forgives all, redeems all, renews all, and unites all. The recognition of mystical unity is not an end in itself; it is redemptive only if it becomes incarnate in the ugly, nitty-gritty, rough-and-tumble of human history. The Gospel demands our engagement in history *now* – for the sake of what lies beyond history. To be so engaged, we have to travel light.

Jesus possessed authority and exercised power over death. He promised, and promises, that if we share his suffering here and now, we share his triumph over the power of death. If we receive our own personal suffering in solidarity with the suffering of the world, then we can present our personal suffering to be transformed into political solidarity and we can experience the gifts of freedom, hope, and joy that such a commitment brings. The sad, pitiful alternative is to turn in on ourselves and ask "Why me?" and live a life of bitterness, complaining, and fear.

We often resist solidarity. Solidarity is uncomfortable. But when we recognize our own helplessness and dependence on the mercy of God – as a critical illness forces us to do – we can experience solidarity and know ourselves as part of the Beloved Community, rooted in God's grace. And then we come to know, without a doubt, that goodness and mercy are doggedly in pursuit of us.

When the most vulnerable among us suffer, we all suffer. This is solid biblical theology, but hardly popular rhetoric in the public arena. Our Grady coalition's message reaffirmed the common good as the most worthy goal of our political action. And I believe the response was so great because we struck a nerve.

On the protest line one day, our good friend Joe Beasley of Concerned Black Clergy and the national leadership of Rainbow Push, commented on the crisis at the pharmacy, "If this had happened at Northside Hospital, they would have called out the National Guard to dispense pills!" Indeed, medical care, prescription drugs, and treatment are guaranteed and readily available for the wealthy, at any cost.

But among the rest of us, many, many people are beginning to understand that we're *all* in trouble. Many middle- and working-class people know that they are paying more and getting less every day. They also know that they live in danger of being unable to get the care deemed necessary by their physicians or of losing insurance coverage altogether. The anxiety is growing right along with the corporate profit margins.

The drive toward privatization will not go away, because human greed is always a part of the human story. But it is never the whole story. The struggle for justice and human dignity is also part of the story. And the struggle heals.

We can move toward a healthier life together when we remember this: A healthy life is possible only when we live with a sense of common good, community, and mutual care. When Dr. Martin Luther King spoke to the marchers who had walked from Selma to Montgomery in 1965, he said, "What we seek is a society at peace with itself." What medicine for our anxiety-ridden nation! Without such a commitment, we live pitted against each other and get sicker and sicker. When we refuse to cooperate with the system that "takes necessities from the masses to give luxuries to the classes," as Dr. King put it, we begin to restore the health of our body politic.

We can have health care – *really good* health care – for every person in the United States of America, of every race, class, gender, and age. We can live together and share the wealth and the good gifts of the land. Until that day comes, we can struggle together to live into the vision. And we'll all get better together.

It is nothing less than a matter of life and death.

Appendix I

SHE

A Poem by Ed Loring

Turmoil
      Tender times too
Scalp Torn.
 Cut
  Split
      Flapped. Grafted. Cow skinned.
Bloody pillow cases
As earliest light tips toes into our room among the catacombs of
memory.

New Top. Old Head.
Beautiful Face.
Blue eyes not yet bleary from time's and cancer's dirty deeds.
Left arm dug deep: skin, flesh, arteries, veins. no bone (bip bam
thank you ma'am)

      like highways paved in
          blood skin
              scarred like Baltimore pot holes.
Thigh stripped
      Skinned like Muley's rabbit strung on barbed wire
Scar like shotgun wound.
Neck sliced
 Arteries veins
  Connected by a master Hindu plumber

Eight hours making connections (from throat to head) with
blood which
    Like breath
      Is Life. (He came to give us Abundant Life).

NOW SHE
  Bleeding ended
  Staples gone
    Swelling
      Like a dead balloon.

SHE
  I say
  Who lies now beside me in the quiet
    Unponcedeleonave   Morning light.
SHE
  Is sleeping like a strong woman readying for the fight for free-
dom's feast

SHE
  Head burnt orange from radiation blasts
    To kill cancer
   To resurrect a healthy head
    Flap baked
     Hair gone
       Won't come back
        Like an abandoned childhood
          Lost.

SHE almost free at last
From the fabulous fickle
  Fingers of cancer. Mr.
   Death's penultimate victory
    Who comes
     Knocks
      Enters
       Flees. Fleeing. Fled.
Once more. (Thank you. Thank you. Thank you. Thank you.
Thank you.)

168

("Because I could not stop for Death
He [unkindly] stopped for me")
SHE
Radiated
  15 times. Five to go.
    Cup full   No: Cup runneth over
      Fire, Earth, Wind, Water.

SHE
    Friday next
    July 14, 2017
a time 72 years ago when the devil danced in New Mexico and
the A Bomb was "tested" and made ready to make ready the end
of God's creation. Japan first (Japs we called them). Who is next?
Will the Korean War ever end? Shall we conquer cancer?

Friday: Crucify Him. Crucify Him
    July 14
    3:20 PM
    Resurrection on the wrong liturgical day
    Down the hall in the Basement (LL2)
    Weinberg Hospital: Johns Hopkins Hospital
      A bell will ding for this SHE.
        But for too many never will the tongue
        Hit the bell curve.

SHE
and I
  Will go home, our new home of splendor and care with St. Francis
standing in
  Front yard surrounded by birds and squirrels to welcome us
HOME.
        Or will we?
            We might stop at the wig store.
And SHE
        Full of life and dancing filled with:
Glory/Thanksgiving/Love/Patience/acceptance/struggle against
the odds

Joyful grandmother gone mad over Michaela's care and playing head-surgery with her dolls and stuffed animals

ME
I say

goddamn the pain
goddamn the suffering
goddamn the bloody pillow case
goddamn the fatigue that locked HER down.
goddamn the weakness of flesh and bone
so in a chair with wheels SHE had, at times,
to
roll.
goddamn the government who will finance the trip to Mercury
and force cancer survivors to run, walk, limp or roll a 5 K Race
for funds for cancer research. goddamn the Republican-Libertarian Party's Health Care (sic) plan which would
have killed HER were she not now old enough for Social Security which is next on
Mitch McConnell's assassination list. And
As in the
WORD
Of one of my Mentors whom Obama denied for votes
Rev. Dr. Jeremiah Wright
"goddamn America."
Knowing Dorothy Day's gentle way:
"Love is the only solution
And Love comes with community."

SHE

Often tells the truthful tale: "Without Hannah here I would have died."

SHE

Nay we, but none like SHE
Is Thankful to our
God who is life force love force
The non-violent Peace Maker

What is Cancer?
      Starving cells
      Cannibals
        Like the Rich eating the Poor
       Sick cells
        Bombing the body like USA drones bomb Syria.
        Drinking the blood
       Eating organs
       Devouring God's children of all ages.
           A singular moment that Death's dutiful Devils
           Don't give a flip about
                You
                Me
                Your Race, sex, gender, religion, nationality,
politics, bank account
       All Cancer wants is
       Our lives.

Thank you God of No War anti-cancer
Thank you Jesus who calls every one of us to
       Healing
Ourselves, our neighbors, our enemies, our earth, our common
good, Syria, Yemen, Palestine, Baltimore, Atlanta and Bamberg.
The whole bunch of us who mess up daily. We are all called to be
Wounded Healers in God's No War fight against cancer and the
military. You
Thank you, Hannah. You are leading us into a deeper life with
your medical skills, your daughter love, your discipleship vocation
as a Wounded Healer: our Nurse among Nurses.

Thank you who have prayed for SHE (and me)
       Sent cards, made calls, composed emails, visited, donated
          YOU in the midst of this mystery named LIFE are es-
sentially Wounded
         Healers in this long haul cancer journey.
Thank you to the Rainbow Women who have cleaned the hospital
floors, scoured the bathroom, changed the sheets, brought laughter
and sharing into the healing arts of making a safe & hygienic space.
Thank you Nurses and doctors: Hindus, Muslims, Jews, Christians,

Atheists, Unknown, African American, African (especially Ibo), White, Brown, Gay, Straight, non-binary (we look forward to the first time we have a transgender nurse or doc)—these folk: The Rainbow of the Wounded Healers—God's creation of diversity. A foretaste of the end of white supremacy and male domination. A glimpse into the wounded healing power of Martin King's call to the Beloved Community.

Thank you to the Board of Directors of the Open Door Community. You worked so hard to make the transition from Atlanta to Baltimore go smoothly. It did not. But your work kept us out of despair and desolation.

> Closing the Open Door Community Atlanta
> Selling our home
> Ah,
> Neo-liberal economics entered the front door of the Presbytery
> While its members railed against the prosperity gospel.
> I Hear the accolades from Milt Friedman reaching up from
> the depths of hell
> With such economic acumen.

> Agape: sacrificial love for others
> Not in style this cycle.

Thank you Martha Murphy Davis (3/5/48). You carried the load and fulfilled W.H. Auden's definition of faith: "To choose what is difficult all one's days, as if it were easy, that is faith."
Thank you Martha Murphy Davis. My Beloved Partner. I adore you. You make accompaniment so light. So easy. Like you, flesh eaten by cancer, enflesh our Lord's "Come unto me all you who labor and are heavy laden. I will give you rest."

Thank you Murphy. How do you do this work? What wondrous love and guts is this? How do you do it? Oh, you make me fall in love with you over and over and over again. I tingle when I touch your thigh scar like a shotgun wound.

Thank you Martha Murphy Davis.

Conclusion One

As I write to you SHE is sleeping, resting, healing, hoping. Building in her dreams another time at bat. And always thankful that she has not struck out.

But...

SHE knows, I know, you know, we know, Jane Keyon knew:

"Someday it will be otherwise."

Yesterday

The two surgeries on her face went very well. The cancer had not spread. Thank you. The Chinese doctor and the white doctor — vibrant women both — and the playful techs worked together. We are deeply grateful. Murphy does have a long incision with many stitches along the side of her face. She lost a little of her ear lobe. The second incision was smaller and less dramatic. At least for me who only stands and waits.

"Joy to the world
All you boy and girls
And all the fishes of the deep blue sea."

Conclusion Two
The Beginning is Near
We began this journey on February 14, 2017 Then:
Friday July 14, 2017
    7 am blood work
    9 am see her hematologist
    10:30 am receive IVIG
    2 pm get the stiches out of her face
    3 pm receive the final blast of radiation
    3:20 pm the bell will ring
    3:25 until death: Free at last. Free at last. Thank God Almighty
she will be
                Free at last.

Love, Ed
July 2017

Appendix II: Resources

Thank you for reading this book!

If you would like to learn more or to journey with the Open Door Community as we serve our sisters and brothers on the streets and in prison, please be in touch. We publish a monthly newspaper, *Hospitality*, which is free, though we appreciate a donation to help with expenses. To subscribe to the paper or learn more, please contact us at:

The Open Door Community
P.O. Box 10980
Baltimore, MD 21234-0980
404-290-2047
opendoorcomm@bellsouth.net
https://www.facebook.com/ODCBalt/
www.opendoorcommunity.org

Our other publications from the Open Door Press include:

Raising Our Voices, Breaking the Chain: The Imperial Hotel Occupation as Prophetic Politics, by Terry Easton (2016)

The Cry of the Poor: Cracking White Male Supremacy — An Incendiary and Militant Proposal, by Eduard Loring (2010)

Sharing the Bread of Life: Hospitality and Resistance at the Open Door Community, by Peter R. Gathje (2006)

A Work of Hospitality: The Open Door Reader 1982-2002, edited by Peter R. Gathje (2002)

I Hear Hope Banging at My Back Door: Writings from Hospitality, by Eduard Loring (2002)

Frances Pauley: Stories of Struggle and Triumph, with an Introduction by Murphy Davis and Foreword by Julian Bond (1996)

Christ Comes in the Stranger's Guise: A History of the Open Door Community, by Peter R. Gathje (1991)

These titles can be ordered from the Open Door Community or downloaded from our website, www.opendoorcommunity.org.